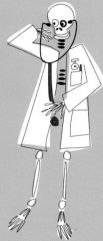

Flesh and Bones of
MEDICAL PHARMACOLOGY

Domenico Spina PhD
Reader in Pharmacology
Sackler Institute of Pulmonary Pharmacology
Pharmaceutical Science Research Division
School of Biomedical and Health Sciences
King's College London
London, UK

Illustrations by Robin Dean

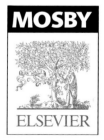

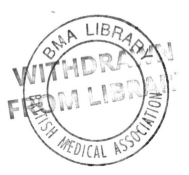

MOSBY
ELSEVIER

Edinburgh   London   New York   Oxford   Philadelphia   St Louis   Sydney   Toronto   2008

MOSBY
ELSEVIER

First published 2008

ISBN-13: 978-0-7234-3353-8

British Library Cataloguing in Publication Data
A catalogue record for this book is available from the British Library

Library of Congress Cataloging in Publication Data
A catalog record for this book is available from the Library of Congress

Notice:
Neither the Publisher nor the Authors assume any responsibility for any loss or injury and/or damage to persons or property arising out of or related to any use of the material contained in this book. It is the responsibility of the treating practitioner, relying on independent expertise and knowledge of the patient, to determine the best treatment and method of application for the patient.
The Publisher

Printed in China

The
publisher's
policy is to use
**paper manufactured
from sustainable forests**

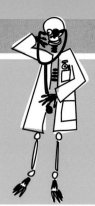

Contents

The big picture

Pharmacology is the study of how chemicals interact with living organisms to produce a biological effect and consequently has a vital role in our understanding of the use of medicines for the treatment and cure of human disease. Pharmacology is concerned with the mechanisms by which chemicals such as neurotransmitters and hormones change body function and this often requires knowledge of many scientific disciplines—chemistry, physiology, biochemistry, immunology and molecular biology. Pharmacology is fundamental for our ability to develop chemicals that may ultimately be used as medicines. There are over 100 'drug' targets and so the magnitude of the task in learning the pharmacology of each drug can seem daunting. To assist in assimilating this information, the student should begin by understanding the mechanisms by which neurotransmitters and hormones alter cell function at the system (i.e. organ) and then cellular (e.g. smooth muscle) levels. This knowledge will help to place in context the rationale for the development and use of different medicines to treat various disorders that affect organ systems, and their associated side-effect profile. The Big Picture should be read first as it gives a basic overview of the nature of drugs, their receptor targets, how drugs are handled by the body, how drugs are developed, and the main body systems affected by drugs.

Pharmacology is the study of the mechanism of action of drugs and consequently involves understanding how drugs work and how their effects are produced. A **drug** is a chemical substance that affects the function of a living organism, but this definition is a little too broad since soap is a chemical that can change function (irritating to the eye). Therefore, it is usual to define a drug as a chemical that is used in a medical context to treat disease and alleviate underlying symptoms. It is also important to recognize that drugs change cell function because they target specific proteins either on or within the cell; these targets are **receptors** (Fig. 1.1), which are sensing proteins that change their activity on binding a drug. It is important to appreciate that binding of a drug to its receptor does not alter the chemical structure of the drug. This may not be the case for chemicals that bind to a target enzyme (e.g. adenylyl cyclase) because they are subject to enzymatic modification (e.g. ATP is converted to cyclic adenosine monophosphate, cAMP).

In general, a chemical is chosen for therapeutic use because it is *specific* for a particular sequence of amino acids within the protein or receptor site, whether this is on the surface of a cell (e.g. cell surface receptor) or within the cell (e.g. an enzyme). Conversely, proteins that act as receptors for endogenous chemicals (or drugs) also show chemical specificity. That is, receptors only recognize substances with a particular chemical structure. The β_2-adrenoceptor demonstrates specificity for epinephrine but not for acetylcholine.

A drug is said to be *selective* if it is found that the chemical interacts with only one receptor family but this can become a little complicated when a receptor family has many subtypes (e.g. α_1, α_2, β_1, β_2, β_3-adrenoceptors). For example, the antihistamine drug **loratidine**, used in the treatment of allergies, is selective for H_1 receptors while the anti-ulcer drug cimetidine is selective for H_2 receptors. Other drugs, such as propranolol, are *non-selective* in the context of binding to β-adrenoceptors; this drug can bind to both β_1- and β_2-adrenoceptors in the β-adrenoceptor family yet it does not bind to α-adrenoceptors. Drugs selectivity is one way of targeting a particular protein while minimizing the possibility of side-effects because of binding to another receptor elsewhere in the body. For example,

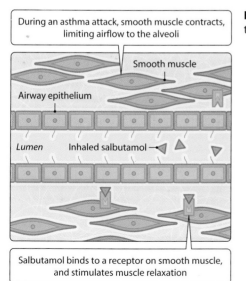

Fig. 1.1 Drugs target receptors.

During an asthma attack, smooth muscle contracts, limiting airflow to the alveoli

Smooth muscle

Airway epithelium

Lumen   Inhaled salbutamol

Salbutamol binds to a receptor on smooth muscle, and stimulates muscle relaxation the anti-epileptic drug chlorpromazine, which is used in the treatment of schizophrenia, binds to dopamine D_2 receptors within the central nervous system (CNS) to produce its anti-psychotic action. However, this drug also produces side-effects, including dry mouth, constipation and blurred vision, because it has a blocking action on muscarinic receptors throughout the body.

■ RECEPTORS

The body releases a wide range of endogenous substances, including neurotransmitters from neuronal cells (e.g. acetyl-choline), hormones (e.g. insulin) or cytokines (e.g. interferon), that alter the function of target cells. In general, a receptor can be defined as a cell macromolecule either on the surface of the cell or within the cytoplasm or nucleus of a cell that is recognized by one of these endogenous substances. The binding of these substances (or drug) to their receptors occurs in a reversible manner involving ionic bonding, hydrogen bonding and van der Waals forces. This initiates a cascade of events that ultimately leads to a change in cell function.

There are four major families of receptors:

■ ligand-gated ion channels (e.g. nicotinic ion channel)
■ G-protein-coupled receptors (e.g. β-adrenoceptor)
■ tyrosine kinase receptors (e.g. insulin receptor)
■ intracellular receptors (e.g. glucocorticosteroid receptor).

These receptors account for a majority of the chemical signalling that occurs within the body and are fundamental to the ability of chemical messengers to alter the function of living cells (Fig. 1.2). Proteins targeted by drugs that do not fall into these four drug receptor families include specific membrane ion pumps (e.g. Na^+/K^+-ATPase), specific enzymes (e.g. 5-phosphodiesterase), structural proteins (e.g. colchicines to tubulin) or cytosolic proteins (e.g. ciclosporin to the immunophilins).

It is important to appreciate that the activation of receptors by chemical substances or drugs is just the first step in altering the function of cells. The activation of receptor leads to a cascade of signalling within the cell involving **second messengers** (e.g. cAMP) that ultimately leads to a biological effect (Fig. 1.3). Any change that affects this cascade can modulate the action of the drug. Nature has provided a system that allows specific interactions between endogenous substances and receptors to regulate the function of cells. Pharmacologists have exploited these specific interactions to develop highly potent and selective chemicals or drugs for the purposes of treating human disease.

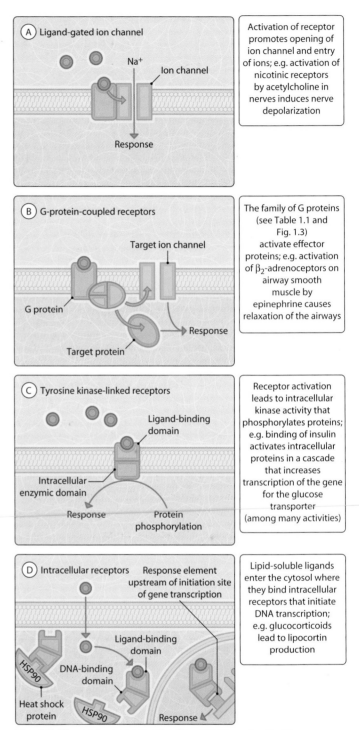

Fig. 1.2 The major receptor families. (A) Ligand-gated ion channels; (B) G-protein-coupled receptors; (C) tyrosine kinase-linked receptors; (D) intracellular receptors.

Drug–receptor interaction

In general, drugs that interact with receptors either mimic the effect of endogenous chemical substances (e.g. neurotransmitters) and are, therefore, referred to as **agonists**, or prevent the action of endogenous chemical substances and are classified as **antagonists**. If agonists and antagonists are to be used as therapeutic agents, they must have a number of important properties.

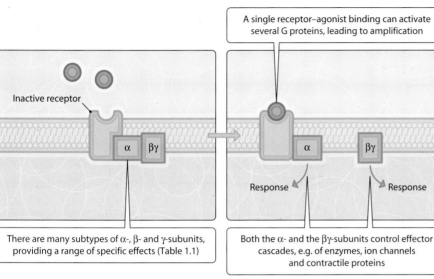

Fig. 1.3 Activation of receptors linked to G proteins, leading to signalling cascades.

Agonists

Agonists associate and dissociate from the target receptor in a reversible manner (Fig. 1.4A). When the rate of association of drug with receptor is equal to the rate of dissociation of this complex, it is understood that the reaction has reached equilibrium. The position of the equilibrium is determined by the concentration of drug and receptor molecules and the **affinity** of drug for its receptor. This affinity is described by the equilibrium **dissociation constant** (K_d) and is a measure of the ability of a drug to bind to its receptor. The higher the affinity (low K_d value) the more likely it is that the receptor will be occupied by drug. Agonists have an additional property called **efficacy**, which is a measure of the ability of an agonist to activate a receptor from its drug-bound (inactive) state. This property explains why some agonists produce maximal responses (**full agonists**) while others only produce submaximal responses (**partial agonists**) in the same target cell. Another class of agonists, called **inverse agonists**, has 'negative efficacy' and produces the opposite effect to agonists.

Often the term **potency** of an agonist is used to give a measure of the biological activity of a drug. In pharmacology, it is usual for a biological response (e.g. contraction of smooth muscle) to be measured (usually in in vitro experiments) with increasing concentrations of an agonist. The effective concentration of

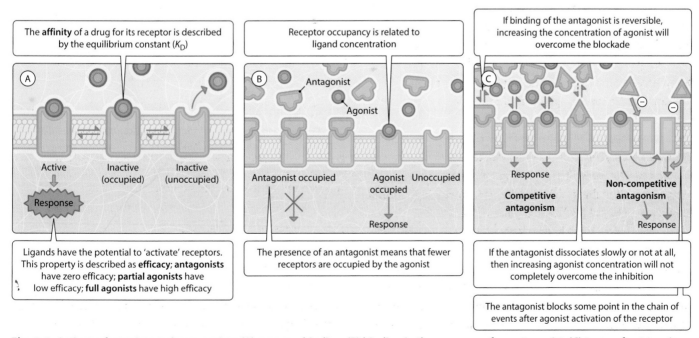

Fig. 1.4 Actions of agonists and antagonists. (A) receptor binding; (B) binding in the presence of an antagonist; (C) types of antagonism.

agonist that produces half-maximal effects (EC_{50}) is a measure of agonist potency. The smaller the value of EC_{50} the more potent is the drug.

Antagonists

Like agonists, antagonists also have affinity for target receptors but differ in one important respect: antagonists do not demonstrate efficacy. As a consequence, antagonists prevent agonists from activating target receptors (Fig. 1.4B). For an antagonist, a measure of its pharmacological **potency** is reflected by the drug's affinity for its receptor, since, by definition, the antagonist has no efficacy. The numerical value for antagonist affinity, the pA_2 ($-\log K_B$) can be derived from a Schild plot and the larger the value the greater the pharmacological potency of the antagonist.

The association and dissociation of antagonist with the receptor is reversible and surmountable by increasing the concentration of competing agonist. This is an example of **competitive antagonism**. Most antagonists used therapeutically are characterized by competitive antagonism (e.g. **propranolol**) and they shift the concentration–response relationship for the agonist to the right but without altering the maximum response. Antagonists that covalently bind to the target site give rise to antagonism that is insurmountable and is, therefore, **irreversible competitive antagonism**.

A developing area of interest that has arisen from experimental observations of receptor binding and activation has suggested that receptors may oscillate between an inactive and activate conformation in the *unoccupied* state. Agonists tend to stabilize the receptor in the active conformation, while inverse agonists stabilize receptors in their inactive states, thereby reducing basal activation of the cell by the unoccupied receptor. Antagonists, by comparison, will bind to both active and inactive conformations of the receptor and prevent the action of agonists. This type of activity is observed using in vitro systems that express abnormally high receptor numbers.

Receptor desensitization

For cells to function normally, the activation of receptors by endogenous chemical substances occurs in a rapid but transient manner. This allows the receptor to return to basal levels of activity ready to be stimulated on a subsequent occasion. However, the continuous exposure of receptor to a drug can give rise to a waning in effectiveness of the drug. This may be a consequence of receptor **desensitization (tachyphylaxis)**. This phenomenon occurs within minutes of receptor activation and provides a homeostatic mechanism to prevent overstimulation of the target cell. Over prolonged periods of repeated drug dosing (days to weeks), pharmacodynamic **tolerance** can develop and this can lead to a reduction in effectiveness of the drug (e.g. repeated administration of opioids).

ADME: ABSORPTION, DISTRIBUTION, METABOLISM AND ELIMINATION

From the preceding discussion, it is clear that it is advantageous for a therapeutic agent to have the characteristic features of *specificity* and *selectivity* of action, which, in general, should lead to improved drugs with fewer side-effects. However, even once an appropriate activity at the selected protein target has been devised, there remain a number of very important considerations that need to be satisfied before the drug is routinely used in patients. The activity and specificity of a drug are determined by its passage into the body, its translocation and metabolism within the body and its elimination from the body. A drug that cannot cross the blood–brain barrier will not cause drowsiness (e.g. a non-sedating antihistamine).

Absorption

There are many ways in which drugs can be introduced into the body, and absorption comprises the processes involved in transferring a drug from the site of administration to the systemic circulation. With the exception of intravenous (i.v.) or intra-arterial administration, a drug needs to cross a cell barrier (e.g. gastrointestinal epithelium) before reaching the systemic circulation. Once in the circulation, the drug needs to cross the capillary wall before reaching extracellular sites in the vicinity of cells and their receptors (Fig. 1.5).

Most drugs in solution exist in equilibrium between their ionized and non-ionized states. The position of this equilibrium is determined by the concentration of both forms of the drug and the **dissociation constant**, K_a (often referred to as pK_a, which is $-\log K_a$). Most drugs are either weak acids or weak

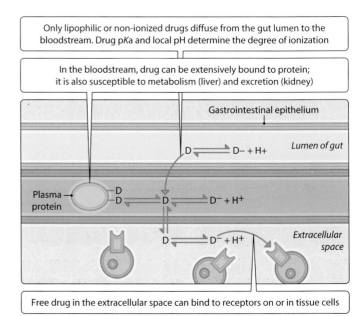

Fig. 1.5 Absorption of drugs.

bases and they can only move across membranes by passive diffusion in their non-ionized lipid-soluble forms. Ionized or polar molecules do not traverse cell membranes by passive diffusion (Fig. 1.5) and the amount of non-ionized drug that diffuses across the membrane will be dependent upon the pH of the aqueous solution. In the stomach, weak acids will exist in their non-ionized forms while weak bases will be ionized; consequently, the environment in the stomach favours absorption of the weak acid. By comparison, increasing the alkalinity of urine will favour the excretion of weak acids, since they will exist in their ionized forms in the urine, thereby preventing reabsorption by the kidney.

The brain has a specialized barrier, known as the **blood–brain barrier**, that prevents polar (ionized) molecules from crossing while non-ionized, lipophilic drugs readily traverse this barrier and gain access to brain interstitial (extracellular) fluid and target sites. However, there are a number of proteins inserted in the membranes of this barrier that act to transport a variety of nutrients in and out of the CNS (e.g. amino acids, glucose). These transporters (e.g. the ATP-binding cassette (ABC) transporters) will also remove drug that has accumulated in the extracellular space back to the systemic circulation. Drugs with low affinity for these transporter systems would be predicted to have a greater distribution within the CNS and this would be a desirable property for a new chemical entity during the development and screening stage for new CNS drugs.

Distribution

Once drug has entered the systemic circulation, it then transfers to the extracellular space of body organs; this process is referred to as distribution. The distribution of drug throughout the body will be dependent upon a number of factors, including blood flow to different organs (e.g. lung high; skin low), lipid solubility of the drug and the extent of plasma protein binding. These are important considerations since it is only free drug that is biologically active and any process that reduces the levels of free drug in the plasma will reduce the concentration of drug within the extracellular compartment and ultimately at receptor sites. For example, circulating drug can be bound in a complex with plasma protein. The amount of drug bound will be dependent upon the affinity constant of the drug for these macromolecules and the presence of other drugs or molecules that could compete for these sites (Fig. 1.5). The binding of a drug to plasma protein (e.g. albumin) has low specificity and does not produce any pharmacological effect, but it does serve to lower the concentration of free drug available to bind to receptor sites and also acts as depot for the drug. The actual concentrations of non-ionized drug in the vicinity of receptor sites will be in equilibrium with free drug in the circulation, but will be considerably smaller than the concentrations bound to plasma protein. As the concentration of drug at receptor sites diminishes (owing to metabolism and/or excretion of drug), so more drug will be 'released' from plasma protein in order to maintain a new equilibrium position.

Metabolism

The body has evolved enzymes that biotransform chemical substances into inactive water-soluble polar molecules; these reactions usually occur in the liver. Most commonly, biotransformation leads to inactivation of pharmacological activity and also produces a more polar metabolite that does not cross the membranes of capillaries in body organs and is readily excreted by the kidney. Occasionally, the drug metabolites may also be pharmacologically active. A **prodrug** is a chemical that is biotransformed to a pharmacologically active metabolite (e.g. conversion of codeine to morphine in the liver).

Orally administered drugs face two problems: the acid environment of the stomach and the blood flow from the gastrointestinal tract to the liver before it reaches the systemic circulation. The acid environment of the stomach can easily inactivate substances such as peptides (e.g. insulin); these must be administered by injection to be effective. An alternative approach is to formulate drugs with coatings (e.g. enteric coating) that protect the drug from destruction in the acid environment of the stomach but break down in the more alkaline intestine. Blood from the gastrointestinal tract is delivered first to the liver; consequently, a drug will be susceptible to biotransformation before it can reach the general circulation. This biotransformation of parent molecule in the liver is commonly referred to as **first-pass metabolism** and can be a major impediment to delivering sufficient quantities of unchanged drug to the systemic circulation. This first-pass metabolism can be avoided by administration of drugs via the inhaled (e.g. salbutamol), intranasal (e.g. vasopressin), buccal (e.g. nitroglycerin) or rectal (e.g. opioids) routes of administration.

The major enzyme family in the liver that metabolizes drugs is the **cytochrome P450 system** (CYP). These enzymes differ in terms of their regulation by inhibitors and inducing agents and in the specificity of their reactions. This family is the major mechanism (but not the only one; alcohol is also metabolized by a cytoplasmic enzyme) of the **phase I reactions**, which are catabolic and act to make the drugs more chemically reactive (e.g. oxidation, deamination, hydroxylation). A second, anabolic, reaction, the **phase 2 reaction**, then conjugates the product to glucuronide or sulphate, giving rise to a more polar molecule that is easier to excrete and is usually inactive. The activity of CYP can be influenced by a number of factors and this must be taken into consideration when administering drugs to patients.

Age, alcohol consumption, smoking and other drugs that are substrates for CYP can either induce or inhibit CYP activity (Fig. 1.6). In humans, there is individual variation in the CYP enzymes, which can have therapeutic significance. For some drugs, the phase I reactions can actually give rise to active drug metabolites; this can be a factor that needs to be taken into account in deciding on drug doses or it can be an effective tool, the inactive prodrug being activated only once absorbed (e.g. biotransformation of bambuterol, which is a carbamate ester of terbutaline).

Elimination

The process of removal of drug from the body occurs by excretion in urine mostly; smaller amounts of drug are excreted in faeces, breast milk, sweat, tears and exhaled air. The kidney is the major site of drug excretion. Blood is filtered in the glomerulus of the kidney by a process that forces plasma fluid through small pores in the glomerular membrane. The filtrate within the renal tubule contains untransformed and non-protein-bound parent drug together with plasma fluid and other small-molecular-weight substances (e.g. carbohydrates). The amount of untransformed drug filtered by this process will depend on how well the drug is bound to protein. Since the transformed drug is more polar, it is not reabsorbed by the kidney and is, therefore, excreted. Untransformed and lipid-soluble drugs may be reabsorbed from the renal tubule back to the circulation and will require biotransformation by the liver

before they are excreted. Transporters present in the renal tubule also promote the excretion of drugs and their metabolites by carrier-mediated elimination (e.g. methotrexate, an acid, and pethidine, a base). Conjugated drugs may also be eliminated by the liver in bile. Once in the intestine, the drug–glucuronide is susceptible to hydrolysis by bacterial enzymes, releasing parent drug that can be reabsorbed into the hepatic portal vein. This leads to what is know as **enterohepatic recycling**.

Assessing the ADME

An understanding of the ADME of drugs is essential for the development of therapeutic drugs but also of practical relevance for administration of drugs to elderly patients (liver dysfunction), children (poorly developed liver) and individuals who have preexisting renal or liver damage. Under these circumstances drug metabolism and elimination from the body must be understood for optimal drug dosing. **Pharmacokinetics** describes how the body deals with a drug: rates of absorption, elimination and distribution of drug throughout the body. It can be examined using mathematical modelling and provides valuable information for determining drug dosing and timing. Of equal importance is a drug's **pharmacodynamics**: what the drug does to the body at its site of action. Together, this information is used by clinicians to decide the appropriate drug dosage (amount plus timing) for a patient. Even armed with these facts, genetic variability within the population will mean that some individuals may not respond to the drug as predicted. A small change (**single nucleotide polymorphism**) of the genetic code can alter the function of proteins. For example, 50% of Caucasians express an enzyme involved in phase 2 reactions that has low enzymatic activity; in such circumstances drugs are acetylated slowly and elimination of the drug will be slower (e.g. procainamide). These individuals are known as slow acetylators. This can have important implications for treating individuals with arrhythmias and who have this polymorphism. Other ethnic groups will have different proportions of slow and fast acetylators. Similarly, genetic variability in the CYP family or transporters can influence the way an individual eliminates a drug. **Pharmacogenetics** is the study of how genetic variability alters the pharmacokinetics and pharmacodynamics of a drug.

■ DRUG EVALUATION

It is a statutory requirement that all drugs intended for use in humans undergo rigorous clinical trials to evaluate drug efficacy and safety. A variety of **preclinical studies** are undertaken in order to evaluate new drug targets and the pharmacology, safety and toxicity of new drugs. This involves a screening process to evaluate newly synthesized molecules on the proposed drug

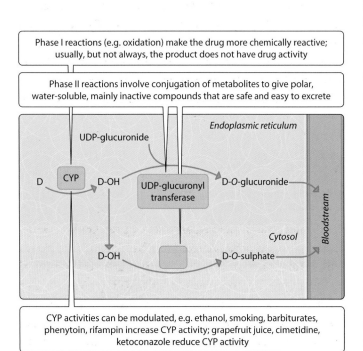

Fig. 1.6 Drug elimination: the cytochrome P450 (CYP) enzyme system.

target using a variety of in vitro assays (human and animal cells). When lead compounds are established, an in vivo evaluation is made in various animal models to obtain information relating to drug efficacy and safety (e.g. mutagenesis, acute toxicity, carcinogenicity and teratogenicity). Once the drug fulfils the necessary criteria of efficacy and safety it is evaluated in human subjects.

Clinical trials

In **phase I clinical trials**, a small group of healthy, usually male, volunteers are administered small doses of drug by the chosen route of administration. Cardiovascular, liver and renal function is monitored for indication of drug toxicity and blood samples are taken to evaluate the pharmacokinetic profile of the drug. In some special circumstances, patients may be used in phase I trials; for example, patients with cancer may be used to evaluate the effect of a potentially novel anticancer drug. In **phase II clinical trials**, groups of patients are used to test the efficacy of the drug. This usually involves a comparison of the efficacy of the drug in several distinct clinical groups (e.g. mild, moderate, severe asthma). These studies also provide information concerning the optimal dose of drug to be used in patients. These trials provide important information concerning how clinically useful the drug may be and whether the chosen drug target is the correct one and, therefore, the drug has a greater probability of succeeding in the next phase of the development. In **phase III clinical trials**, a detailed understanding of the pharmacodynamic properties of the drug in patients is obtained. It is usual for patients to be randomized to receive either placebo or drug (the drug may be compared with either placebo or an existing medication for the condition). It is also usual for the subject and investigator to be unaware of which treatment is being given and the trial is then known as a double-blind study. The biological marker(s) of drug efficacy are monitored before and then during the treatment arm of the trial. Side-effects of drug treatment are also monitored regularly. **Phase IV** or **postmarketing surveillance** is used to detect unexpected, rare or long-term adverse effects that might arise once the drug is available for prescription to the wider patient community.

Adverse reaction to drugs

Adverse reaction to drugs can either be predictable based on an understanding of the pharmacology of the drug or be unpredictable/idiosyncratic. For example, drowsiness caused by some antihistamines used for the treatment of allergies is caused by H_1 receptor blockade in the CNS and is predictable, as is excess bleeding with an anticoagulant. This type of reaction is know as a **type A** adverse drug reaction. In some circumstances, an adverse reaction not anticipated from the pharmacology of

the drug may arise but is predictable if the drug is consumed in large doses (e.g. paracetamol toxicity in the liver). Some adverse events occur with normal drug dosage and are unpredictable and uncommon (e.g. agranulocytosis with carbimazole; anaphylaxis with penicillin). Rare adverse events that are unknown or idiosyncratic are referred to as **type B** adverse drug reactions.

The liver is a major site of biotransformation; consequently, there is a possibility that some drugs might form reactive metabolites. Of these, some may be useful and others harmful (e.g. cyclophosphamide produces first the active metabolite phosphoramide mustard and then the toxic metabolite acrolein). These reactive species can covalently bind to proteins, lipids, carbohydrates or DNA, which can lead to cell toxicity and death. The liver and kidney are particularly susceptible to this type of toxicity. For example, paracetamol is converted by CYP to a reactive species that binds covalently to cell macromolecules, leading to cell necrosis. Normally this reactive species is conjugated with glutathione in the liver to give an inactive polar metabolite that is excreted by the kidney. Overdose with paracetamol leads to depletion of liver glutathione levels, which leaves the hepatocyte susceptible to cell damage by these reactive species and **hepatoxicity** ensues. Reactive metabolites can also be cytotoxic by non-covalent mechanisms (e.g. generation of toxic oxygen radicals). Other drugs causing hepatotoxicity include methotrexate and isoniazid.

If drugs or their metabolites interact with DNA, they can cause **mutagenesis** and **carcinogenesis**. This is usually the result of covalent modification of DNA and the inability of the cell to arrest cell cycle progression during mitosis. Cytotoxic drugs used in cancer therapy have the potential to be mutagenic. Other drugs (e.g. thalidomide, cytotoxic drugs, retinoids and anti-epileptic drugs) induce structural malformations in the growing fetus and are referred to as **teratogenic**. These drugs must be avoided during pregnancy.

A number of drugs are known to cause **immunological adverse reactions**, which are the most common form of adverse reaction. Drugs are usually too small to stimulate the immune system on their own but they can act as **haptens**, forming complexes with cell components that are capable of stimulating the immune system, causing adverse drug reactions. In **type I** immediate or anaphylactic reactions, the binding of hapten to IgE-bearing mast cells causes activation and release of histamine, prostaglandins and leukotrienes from these cells. The result is bronchoconstriction, hypotension, swelling of soft tissue and urticaria. Systemic administration of penicillin can induce anaphylactic shock in susceptible individuals and can be life threatening. In **type II** cytotoxic reactions, interaction of drug with cell components recognized by IgG activates complement and causes cell lysis. Haemolytic anaemia (penicillin, methyldopa), thrombocytopenia (digitoxin) and neutropenia (phenylbutazone) can cause adverse drug reactions in certain individuals. In **type III reactions**, or immune-complex reaction, drug–protein complexes are deposited on basement membranes of endothelial cells giving rise to a local inflammatory response. In **type IV** or delayed-type hypersensitivity reaction, the drug complex stimulates the recruitment of T lymphocytes and gives rise to localized inflammation. In the skin, this leads to irritation and oedema, manifested clinically as a skin rash. Drug-induced haematological reactions, destroying both formed elements in the circulation and progenitor cells in bone marrow, can be caused by types II–IV hypersensitivity. Such reactions lead to haemolytic anaemia (e.g. methyldopa), loss of leukocytes (agranulocytosis, e.g. clozapine) or thrombocytopenia (e.g. heparin)—or even loss of all lineages (aplastic anaemia, e.g. chloramphenicol).

Drug interactions

Many patients, but particularly the elderly, will be receiving more than one medication, either for the treatment of different diseases or for the same disease. Hence the potential for drug interaction is considerable. The interaction may result in a decrease in effectiveness of the drug response or might increase the clinical response. This can be predicted by the **pharmacodynamics** of the different medications. For example, β_2-agonists and glucocorticosteroids are often used together in the treatment of asthma. The bronchodilatation caused by a β_2-agonist may be enhanced because glucocorticosteroids can increase the synthesis of β_2-adrenoceptors. Monoamine oxidase inhibitors prevent the destruction of norepinephrine in noradrenergic neurons and will enhance the actions of tyramine (contained in cheese) on sympathetic neurons (throbbing headache); in this case, an adverse drug reaction is caused.

Drug interactions can also occur through changes in the **pharmacokinetics** of the drug. Ascorbic acid facilitates the transport of ferric ions across the gastrointestinal epithelium, while metoclopromide (used to hasten gastric emptying in patients with gastro-oesophageal reflux), will accelerate gastrointestinal absorption of another drug. In contrast, opioids tend to reduce gastric motility and thereby slow the rate of absorption of drugs. Drug binding to plasma proteins may be susceptible to displacement by a competing drug (e.g. phenytoin and aspirin).

The activity of the major biotransforming enzymes (CYP) in the liver can be altered by drugs. The metabolism of theophylline is increased by drugs that induce CYP activity (e.g. barbiturates, phenytoin) and reduced by drugs that inhibit CYP activity (e.g. cimetidine, oral contraceptives). This interaction will alter the clinical effectiveness of the drug and could lead to an increase in drug side-effects. The excretion of one drug can also be affected by another. Probenecid is an example of a drug specifically designed to prevent the excretion of penicillin by the kidney. Probenecid inhibits organic anion transporters in the renal tubules, thereby preventing the excretion of penicillin.

■ MAIN BODY SYSTEMS

The function of living cells is regulated by numerous chemical signals including neurotransmitters (e.g. acetylcholine), hormones (e.g. glucocorticosteroids), lipid mediators (e.g. prostaglandins), blood elements (e.g. coagulation system) and small-molecular-weight proteins (e.g. cytokines). The ability to develop novel therapeutics to treat diseases depends on an understanding of the mechanism by which these chemical substances interact with cells, or an understanding of the underlying pathology of the disease process and how this affects cell function. In order to begin to understand how drugs work at an organ or system level, it is necessary first to understand the physiological regulation of the different organ systems.

Autonomic nervous system

The peripheral nervous system regulates the function of all of the body organs and includes the cranial and spinal nerves and the autonomic nervous system (Fig. 1.7). The autonomic nervous system, as the name suggests, is outside voluntary control, but nonetheless is derived from the CNS and, therefore, cannot function in its absence. It has two subdivisions, the **parasympathetic** and the **sympathetic** systems (Fig. 1.8); these systems use acetylcholine and norepinephrine as neurotransmitters, respectively. The adrenal medulla, which is part of the sympathetic nervous system, releases a hormone, epinephrine. These neurotransmitters can alter the function of cells in a precise and coordinated fashion. It is often convenient, but a gross oversimplification, to view the parasympathetic nervous system in the context of regulating the body at rest ('rest and digest'), while the sympathetic nervous system prepares the body for physical exertion ('flight and fright'). Anatomically, the parasympathetic and sympathetic nervous systems consist of two neurons separated by a synapse (Fig. 1.9). This synapse occurs in an autonomic ganglion outside the CNS. In contrast, a single motor neuron connects the CNS with skeletal muscle in the somatic efferent system (Fig. 1.9). In general, parasympathetic ganglia are located within the organs, with the exception of the head and neck, while sympathetic ganglia are found on either side of the spinal column (Figs 1.7 and 1.9).

Both the parasympathetic and the sympathetic systems are important in regulating cell function under physiological conditions and while there are many examples where they have opposing action it is better to consider each as having their own

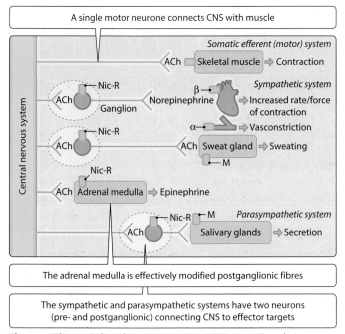

Fig. 1.7 The peripheral nervous system. NE, norepinephrine; ACh, acetylcholine; Nic-R, nicotinic receptor; β, β-adrenoceptor; α, α-adrenoceptor; M, muscarinic receptor.

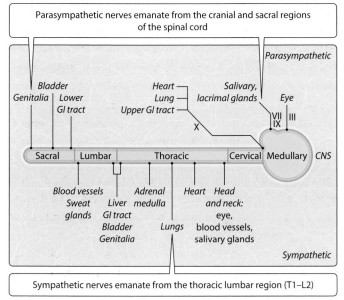

Fig. 1.8 Basic plan of the autonomic nervous system.

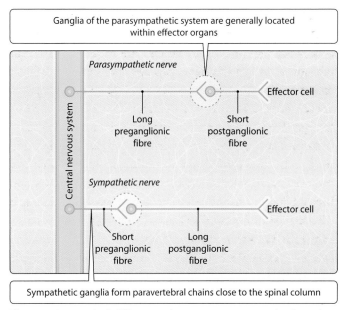

Fig. 1.9 Anatomical differences between parasympathetic and sympathetic systems.

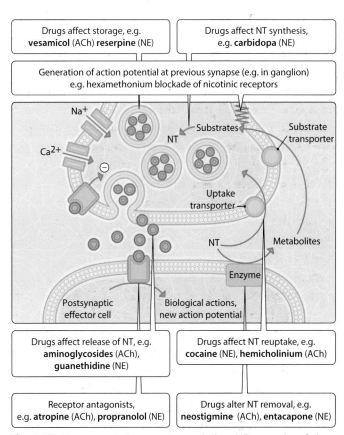

Fig. 1.10 Drug targets in neurotransmission. NE, norepinephrine; ACh, acetylcholine; NT, neurotransmitter.

effect on cell function. These two systems regulate cell function by releasing neurotransmitters that stimulate a biological response by activating receptors on postsynaptic membranes (Fig. 1.10).

The synthesis, storage, release and removal of neurotransmitter within the neuroeffector junction are potential targets for a number of therapeutic agents (Fig. 1.10). For example, carbidopa prevents the conversion of levodopa to dopamine within peripheral sympathetic nerve terminals, which ensures

that more levodopa is available for conversion to dopamine within the CNS for the treatment of Parkinson's disease. Activation of presynaptic α_2-adrenoceptors on sympathetic neurons reduces the release of norepinephrine from nerve terminals and, therefore, clonidine is used in the treatment of hypertension. Alternatively, inhibition of postsynaptic β-adrenoceptors prevents activation of cardiac muscle and provides a rationale basis for the use of propranolol in the treatment of hypertension (see Fig. 1.13, below).

Endocrine system

Hormones including insulin, thyroid hormone, sex hormone and adrenal corticosteroids regulate cell growth, differentiation and cell homeostasis; drugs targeting these systems have therapeutic utility (Table 1.1). Hormones bind to receptors in

Table 1.1 SOME EXAMPLES OF DRUGS AND THEIR USE IN ENDOCRINOLOGICAL CONDITIONS

Agent/drug	Molecular target	Effect on target	Clinical effect	Condition
Pancreas				
Insulin	Insulin receptor	Agonist	Promotes glucose uptake	Type I diabetes
Glibenclamide	ATP-sensitive K channel	Inhibitor	Promotes insulin secretion	Type II diabetes
Repaglinide	ATP-sensitive K channel	Inhibitor	Promotes insulin secretion	Type II diabetes
Rosiglitazone	Peroxisome proliferators-activated receptor gamma (PPARγ)	Agonist	Increase insulin sensitivity and lower blood glucose levels	Type II diabetes
Thyroid gland				
Thioureylenes (carbimazole)	Thyroid peroxidase	Inhibits	Inhibits thyroxine synthesis	Graves' disease
Thyroxine	Thyroid receptor	Stimulates	Mimics the effect of the natural hormone	Deficiency disorders (e.g. Hashimoto's thyroiditis)
Sex hormones				
Buserelin, goserelin	Gonadotrophin receptors	Agonist	Stimulates (pulsatile) gonadotrophin receptors	Infertility
			Downregulates (chronic) gonadotrophin receptors	Breast cancer
Oestrogens	ER	Agonist	Replenish endogenous oestrogens	Hormone replacement therapy
Ethinylestradiol/progestin	ER/progestogen receptor	Agonist	Suppresses release of follicle-stimulating hormone and luteinizing hormone	Oral contraception
Clomiphene	ER (pituitary)	Antagonist	Stimulates gonadotrophin release	Infertility
Anastrozole	Aromatase enzyme	Inhibitor	Prevents oestrogen formation	Breast cancer
Tamoxifen	ERα, ERβ	Partial agonist	Inhibits oestrogen signalling	Breast cancer
Raloxifene	ERα, ERβ	Partial agonist (ERα), antagonist (ERβ)	Inhibits oestrogen signalling	Osteoporosis
Finasteride	5α-reductase enzyme (type II)	Inhibitor	Inhibits conversion of testosterone to dihydrotestosterone	BHP
Cyproterone	Androgen receptor	Partial agonist	Inhibits androgen signalling	BHP, prostate cancer
Flutamide	Androgen receptor	Antagonist	Inhibits androgen signalling	BHP, prostate cancer
Trilostane	3β-Hydroxysteroid dehydrogenase	Inhibitor	Inhibits the formation of glucocorticosteroids and mineralcorticosteroids	Cushing's syndrome, prostate cancer, acne in women, hirsutism
Adrenal hormones				
Hydrocortisone	Corticosteroid receptor	Agonist	Replenishes endogenous corticosteroid activity	Addison's disease
Glucocorticosteroids (budesonide, prednisolone)	Glucocorticosteroid receptor	Agonist	Anti-inflammatory	Asthma, rheumatoid arthritis
Fludrocortisone	Mineralcorticosteroid receptor	Agonist	Replenishes endogenous mineralcorticosteroid activity (Na$^+$ reabsorption, fluid retention)	Addison's disease, hypoaldosteronism

ER, oestrogen receptor; BHP, benign prostatic hyperplasia.

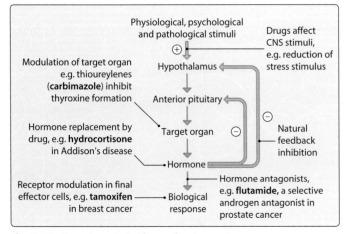

Fig. 1.11 Drug targets in the endocrine system.

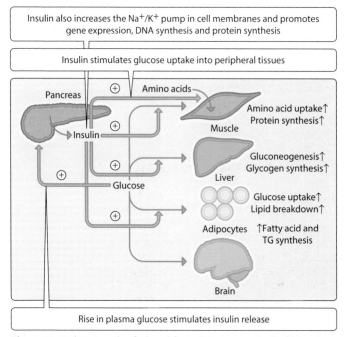

Fig. 1.12 Balancing the fed and fasted states: control of blood glucose. TG, triacylglycerol.

target cells and induce a biological response. Hydrophilic ligands such as insulin act in a similar way to neurotransmitters by binding to receptors on the cell surface. These receptors have integral enzyme activity, belonging to the family of tyrosine kinase receptors (insulin). Once activated, these receptors can rapidly alter cellular activity via second messenger cascades but can also alter gene transcription, with less-rapid results. Lipophilic ligands, such as thyroid hormone, sex hormones and adrenal corticosteroids, enter the cell and bind to intracellular receptors. Once activated, these drug–receptor complexes move to the nucleus and initiate changes in the rate of gene transcription and the synthesis of biologically important proteins. Biological responses to cell surface receptors can occur within seconds; biological responses to intracellular receptors occur in minutes to hours.

Clinically useful drugs have been developed to mimic the actions of endogenous hormone in deficiency disorders or to inhibit the activity of the hormone in situations where persistent stimulation is undesirable (Fig. 1.11). Drugs can have beneficial actions by targeting hormone synthesis, release or endogenous actions. The most common endocrine disorder is **diabetes mellitus**, which has wide-ranging effects that reflect the central role of insulin in metabolic balance (Fig. 1.12).

Central nervous system

The CNS comprises the brain and spinal cord and controls motor function, the autonomic nervous system and the endocrine system. The CNS is an extremely complex network of interconnecting neuronal pathways. Each neuron comprises a cell body (soma) and an axon, which forms a connection or synapse to a postsynaptic cell. The cell bodies also have neural projections (dendrites) that can terminate on the cell body itself, on the cell body of another nerve or on the presynaptic terminal

of a third neuron that is making a neuronal connection to a postsynaptic cell (Fig. 1.13). It is, therefore, not surprising that a number of different neurotransmitter systems are involved in neuronal communication within the CNS.

Some examples of important neurotransmitters within the brain include γ-**aminobutyric acid** (**GABA**), **glutamate** and **dopamine**. GABA is synthesized from glutamate and stored in vesicles in the terminal endings of GABAergic neurons. It is the major inhibitory neurotransmitter within the CNS (Fig. 1.13). GABA activates $GABA_A$ receptors, which leads to Cl^- entry and cell hyperpolarization, thereby reducing postsynaptic neuronal excitability and neurotransmitter release by the postsynaptic neuron. Clinically relevant drugs include the benzodiazepines (e.g. diazepam), which target $GABA_A$ receptors and enhance the action of GABA. Theses are used as anxiolytic, sedative and anticonvulsant drugs. Glutamate is one of the most abundant excitatory neurotransmitters in the brain. It is synthesized from glutamine and stored in vesicles within the terminal endings of the glutaminergic neurons (Fig. 1.13). Glutamate released from these nerve terminals can activate a number of postsynaptic receptors including the AMPA and NMDA receptors (so-called because they are activated by the agonists α-amino-3-hydroxy-5-methyl-4-isoxazolepropionic acid and N-methyl-D-asparate, respectively). The entry of Na^+ and Ca^{2+} into the postsynaptic neuron causes membrane depolarization and increases cell excitability. Drugs like ketamine block NMDA receptors and are

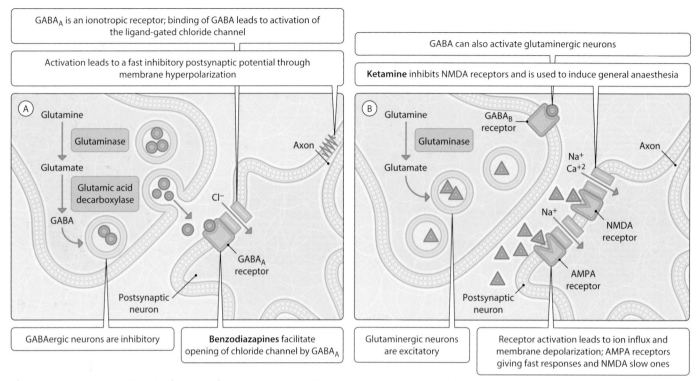

Fig. 1.13 Neurotransmitters in the central nervous system. (A) GABAergic neurons; (B) glutaminergic neurons.

used as general anaesthetics. Other examples of neurotransmitters and drugs that target the activity of these systems in clinical conditions are summarized in Table 1.2.

Peripheral organ systems

A number of clinically effective drugs work by mimicking or interfering with the actions of endogenous chemical substances or processes to elicit the desired biological response, but these are too numerous to describe here. It is important to keep in mind the big picture of how each organ system is regulated by

endogenous chemical substances/processes in order to appreciate the rationale for the use of therapeutic drugs. For example, there are many diseases that affect the cardiovascular system and these may affect the heart itself, the vascular system, the kidneys and so on (e.g. hypertension, angina pectoris, arrhythmias, congestive heart disease, renal failure). These effects can be ameliorated by targeting the actual malfunction (e.g. anti-arrhythmic drugs) or by altering the system as a whole (e.g. use of diuretics). Figure 1.14 (p. 15) summarizes the drugs and their targets in cardiovascular disease. The different drug classes have

Table 1.2 EXAMPLES OF DRUGS THAT ALTER CHEMICAL NEUROTRANSMISSION WITHIN THE CENTRAL NERVOUS SYSTEM

Neurotransmitter and clinical condition	Drug	Molecular target	Effect on target	Clinical effect
Dopamine Parkinson's disease	Levodopa	Dopaminergic neurons in the substantia nigra	Agonist	Replenishes diminishing dopamine content within basal ganglia
	Carbidopa	Dopa decarboxylase	Inhibitor	Prevents conversion of levodopa to dopamine in peripheral nerve terminals
	Apomorphine, bromocriptine, pergolide, ropinirole	D receptor	Agonist	Inhibit GABAergic activity to the thalamus and stimulate movement (mimic dopamine)
	Selegiline	MAOB	Inhibitor	Prolongs the duration of action

Table 1.2 EXAMPLES OF DRUGS THAT ALTER CHEMICAL NEUROTRANSMISSION WITHIN THE CENTRAL NERVOUS SYSTEM—Cont'd

Neurotransmitter and clinical condition	Drug	Molecular target	Effect on target	Clinical effect
	Entacapone	Catecholamine-O-methyltransferase	Inhibitor	of levodopa by preventing metabolism of dopamine Prolongs the duration of levodopa by preventing removal of dopamine from extraneuronal sites
Nausea and vomiting	Domperidone, metoclopromide	D_2 receptors	Antagonist	Inhibit dopaminergic stimulation of the chemoreceptor trigger zone
Antipsychotics (schizophrenia)	Haloperidol, perphenazine, chlorpromazine	D_2 receptors	Antagonist	Inhibit dopaminergic overactivity in the mesolimbic system (reduces positive symptoms) and promote dopaminergic activity in the mesocortical system (reduces negative symptoms)
GABA				
Anxiolytic, sedative, hypnotic uses	Diazepam, midazolam, temazepam	$GABA_A$ receptor	Agonist	Enhance opening of $GABA_A$ (ω_{1-3} subtypes) receptors by GABA, facilitating chloride entry, membrane hyper-polarization and reduced neuronal excitability
Hypnotic (insomnia)	Zopiclone, zolidem	$GABA_A$ receptors	Agonist	As above; show selectivity for $GABA_A$ (ω_1 subtype) receptor and reduce excitability of nerves
Anti-epileptic	Clonazepam, diazepam	$GABA_A$ receptors	Agonist	Second-line therapy in partial and generalized seizures
	Vigabatrin	GABA transaminase	Inhibitor	Prevents the inactivation of GABA
	Tiagabine	GABA transporter	Inhibitor	Prevents reuptake of GABA
Antispastic	Baclofen	$GABA_B$ receptor	Agonist	Activation of these G-protein-coupled receptors leads to reduced neurotransmitter release and reduces excitability of spinal neurons
General anaesthetics	Inhalational: halothane, nitrous oxide; intravenous: propofol, etomidate	$GABA_A$ receptors	Agonist	Enhance $GABA_A$-mediated inhibitory responses
	Ketamine (intravenous)	NMDA receptor	Antagonist	Inhibits NMDA-mediated excitation
Serotonin (5HT)				
Anxiolytics	Buspirone	Presynaptic $5HT_{1A}$ receptor	Partial agonist	Hyperpolarization of raphe 5HT neurons, reducing excitability (acute) but anxiolysis occurs after days to weeks suggesting complex action on neuronal plasticity
Antipsychotic	Clozapine, risperidone, sertindole	$5HT_{2A}$, $5HT_{2C}$ receptors	Antagonist	Inhibition of 5HT receptors in the cortex contributes toward their clinical effect
Antidepressants	Tricyclic drugs (imipramine, doxepine)	5HT and norepinephrine transporter	Inhibitor	Inhibition of 5HT transporter increases the availability of 5HT at pre- and postsynaptic receptors
	Citalopram, fluoxetine, paroxetine	5HT transporter	Inhibitor	As above

Continued

Table 1.2 EXAMPLES OF DRUGS THAT ALTER CHEMICAL NEUROTRANSMISSION WITHIN THE CENTRAL NERVOUS SYSTEM—Cont'd

Neurotransmitter and clinical condition	Drug	Molecular target	Effect on target	Clinical effect
	Venlafaxine	5HT and norepinephrine transporter	Inhibitor	As above
	Mirtazapine	$5HT_{2A}$ receptor	Antagonist	Inhibits $5HT_{2A}$ receptor activity (cortex, hippocampus)
	Trazodone	$5HT_{2C}$ receptors	Antagonist	Inhibits $5HT_{2C}$ receptor activity (cortex, hippocampus)
	Phenelzine, tranylcypromine	MAOA/B	Inhibitor	Irreversible inhibition of these enzymes prevents degradation of 5HT; so more is available for release
	Moclobemide	MAOA	Inhibitor	Reversible and selective inhibitor of MAOA
Nausea and vomiting	Ondansetron	$5HT_3$ receptor	Antagonist	$5HT_3$ receptor antagonism in chemoreceptor trigger zone (CTZ)
Migraine	Sumatriptan	$5HT_{1B/1D}$ receptor	Agonist	Agonist that stimulates vasoconstriction of meningeal vessels, inhibits neuropeptide release from, and excitability of, sensory nerves
Norepinephrine (noradrenaline) Antidepressants	Tricyclic drugs (imipramine, doxepine)	5HT and norepinephrine transporter	Inhibitor	Inhibition of the norepinephrine transporter increases the availability of norepinephrine at pre- and postsynaptic receptors
	Phenelzine, tranylcypromine	MAOA,B	Inhibitor	Irreversible inhibition of these enzymes prevents degradation of norepinephrine in nerves, making more available for release
	Moclobemide	MAOA	Inhibitor	Reversible and selective inhibitor of MAOA
	Venlafaxine	5HT and norepinephrine transporter	Weak Inhibitor	As tricyclic drugs
	Reboxetine	Norepinephrine transporter	Inhibitor	Increased availability of norepinephrine at pre- and postsynaptic receptors
	Mirtazapine	Presynaptic α_2-adrenoceptor; postsynaptic $5HT_2$, $5HT_3$ receptors	Antagonist at all	Inhibition of presynaptic inhibitory influence on noradrenergic and serotonergic nerves
Opioid Analgesic	Morphine, codeine, fentanyl	Opioid μ receptors	Agonist	Inhibit excitatory neurotransmission in nociceptor pathway
Acetylcholine (cholinergic) Alzheimer's disease	Donazepil, rivastigmine, tacrine	Acetycholinesterase	Inhibitor	Promote cholinergic neurotransmission involved in memory and learning
Parkinson's disease	Benztropine	Muscarinic receptor	Antagonist	Interferes with cholinergic neurotransmission in the striatum thereby promoting movement

GABA; γ-aminobutyric acid; MAO, monamine oxidase.

been developed based on an understanding of the mechanisms that regulate the function of the heart, circulation and kidney. In hypertension, blood pressure can be reduced by selective blockade of β-adrenoceptors (beta-blockers, e.g. propranolol), reduction of sympathetic drive (clonidine), increasing vascular dilatation (nitrovasodilators), interference with the renin–angiotensin system (angiotensin-converting enzyme (ACE) inhibitors, e.g. captopril; angiotensin II receptor antagonists, e.g. losartan) or reduction of blood volume (diuretics, e.g. thiazides). Selected examples of drugs that target receptors in different body organs in the treatment of various clinical conditions are summarized in Table 1.3.

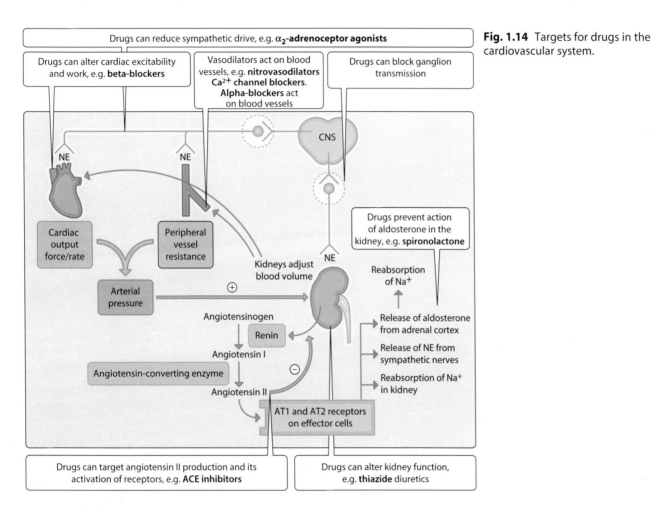

Fig. 1.14 Targets for drugs in the cardiovascular system.

Table 1.3 EXAMPLES OF DRUGS THAT AFFECT BODY ORGANS

Agent/drug	Molecular target	Effect on target	Clinical effect	Condition
Respiratory tract				
Salbutamol	β_2-Adrenoceptor	Agonist	Bronchodilatation	Asthma, COPD
Ipratropium bromide	Muscarinic receptor	Antagonist	Bronchodilatation	Asthma, COPD
Fluticasone propionate	Glucocorticosteroid receptor	Agonist	Anti-inflammatory	Asthma
Montelukast	Cysteinyl-leukotriene 1 receptor	Antagonist	Bronchoprotection (weak anti-inflammatory)	Asthma
Xanthines	Phosphodiesterase	Inhibitor	Bronchodilator/anti-inflammatory	Asthma, COPD
Cromoglycate	Unknown	Inhibition	Weak anti-inflammatory	Asthma
Gastrointestinal tract				
Cimetidine	H_2 receptor	Antagonist	Inhibits acid secretion	Peptic ulcers
Ompremazole	H^+/K^+-ATPase	Inhibitor	Inhibits acid secretion	Peptic ulcers

Continued

Table 1.3 EXAMPLES OF DRUGS THAT AFFECT BODY ORGANS—Cont'd

Agent/drug	Molecular target	Effect on target	Clinical effect	Condition
Loperamide	Opioid μ receptor	Agonist	Antimotility, antisecretory	Diarrhoea
Ondansetron	Serotonin $5HT_3$ receptor	Antagonist	Inhibits nerve activity	Anti-emetic
Metoclopromide	Serotonin 5HT receptor, dopamine D_2 receptor	Antagonist	Inhibits nerve activity	Anti-emetic
Domperidone	Dopamine D_2 receptor	Antagonist	Inhibits nerve activity	Anti-emetic
Renal system				
Loop diuretic (furosemide)	$Na^+/K^+/2Cl^-$ transporter	Inhibitor	Na^+ loss, diuresis	Hypertension, oedema, (CHF, nephritic syndrome, hepatic cirrhosis)
Thiazide diuretic (hydrochlorothiazide)	Na^+/Cl^- transporter	Inhibitor	Na^+ loss, diuresis	Hypertension
Spironolactone	Aldosterone receptor	Antagonist	Reduces synthesis/activity of sodium transporters/channels	CHF, primary hyperaldosteronism
Amiloride	Sodium channels	Channel blocker	Na^+ loss, diuresis	As above
Urogenital system				
Tolterodine	Muscarinic M_3 receptor	Antagonist	Decreases bladder activity	Urinary incontinence
Tamsulosin	α_1-Adrenoceptor	Antagonist	Inhibits contraction of prostate and bladder neck smooth muscle	BPH
Finasteride	5α-Reductase enzyme (type II)	Inhibitor	Inhibits formation of dihydrotestosterone	BPH
Sildenafil	Phosphodiesterase 5	Inhibitor	Smooth muscle dilatation	Erectile dysfunction
Alprostadil	Prostaglandin receptor	Agonist	Smooth muscle dilatation	Erectile dysfunction
Terbutaline	β_2-Adrenoceptor	Agonist	Uterine relaxation	Tocolytic (prevents premature birth)
Eye				
Timolol	β-Adrenoceptor	Antagonist	Inhibits aqueous humour formation	Open-angle glaucoma
Acetazolamide	Carbonic anhydrase	Inhibitor	Inhibits aqueous humour formation	Open-angle glaucoma
Brimonidine	α_2-Adrenoceptor	Agonist	Inhibits aqueous humour formation	Open-angle glaucoma
Pilocarpine	Muscarinic receptor	Agonist	Stimulates drainage	Open-angle glaucoma
Latanoprost	Prostaglandin $F_{2\alpha}$ receptor	Agonist	Stimulates drainage	Open-angle glaucoma
Tropicamide	Muscarinic receptor	Agonist	Pupil dilatation (mydriasis)	Ophthalmological examination
Phenylephrine	α-Adrenoceptor agonist	Agonist	Pupil dilatation, vasoconstriction	Allergic conjunctivitis
Azelastine	Histamine H_1 receptor	Antagonist	Reduces vascular oedema	Allergic conjunctivitis
Skin				
Benzoyl hydroxide	Bacteria		Bacteriocidal	Acne
Azelaic acid	Cytochrome P450 reductase, bacteria, virus	Inhibitor, antibacterial, antiviral	Inhibits DNA synthesis in keratinocytes	Acne
Isotretinoin	Retinoic acid receptor	Agonist	Comedolytic	Acne
Antibiotics	Bacteria		Kill bacteria	Acne
Coal tar	DNA	Cross-links DNA	Cytostatic	Psoriasis
Tazarotene, acitretin	Retinoic acid receptor	Agonist	Anti-inflammatory, cytostatic	Psoriasis
Calcipotriene	Vitamin D receptor	Agonist	Immunosuppressant, regulates epidermal proliferation	Psoriasis
Phototherapy and psoralen	DNA	DNA intercalation	Inhibits DNA synthesis (lymphocytes and epidermal cells)	Psoriasis
Ciclosporin	Calcineurin	Inhibitor	Immunosuppressant	Psoriasis, atopic dermatitis

Table 1.3 EXAMPLES OF DRUGS THAT AFFECT BODY ORGANS—Cont'd

Agent/drug	Molecular target	Effect on target	Clinical effect	Condition
Methotrexate	Dihydrofolate reductase	Inhibitor	Antifolate; inhibition of DNA synthesis (immunosuppressant, cytostatic)	Psoriasis, atopic dermatitis
Fluticasone propionate	Glucocorticosteroid receptor	Agonist	Anti-inflammatory	Atopic dermatitis
Liver				
Statins (simvastatin, pravastatin)	Hydroxymethyl-glutamyl-CoA reductase	Inhibitor	Inhibits formation of cholesterol in the liver	Dyslipidaemia
Bile-binding resins (colestyramine)	Bile salts	Chemical inactivation	Reduced reabsorption of excreted bile (cholesterol depletion in the liver)	Dyslipidaemia
Fibrates (bezafibrate, gemfibrozil)	Peroxisome proliferator-activated receptor-α	Agonist	Increases free fatty acid uptake into tissues, lipoprotein lipase activity and plasma high density lipoprotein	Dyslipidaemia
Cardiovascular system: heart and vessels				
Lidocaine (class I)	Sodium channels	Inhibitor	Reduces cardiac excitability	Arrhythmia
Beta-blockers (atenolol) (class II)	β-Adrenoceptor	Antagonist	Slows SA node activity	Arrhythmia
Amiodarone (class III)	Potassium, sodium, calcium channels	Inhibitor	Prolongs Q-T interval	Arrhythmia
Verapamil (class IV)	L-type calcium channels	Inhibitor	Slows conduction in SA and AV node	Arrhythmia
Glyceryl trinitrate	Guanylyl cyclase	NO donor (activator)	Smooth muscle relaxation	Angina
Beta-blockers	β-Adrenoceptors	Inhibitor	Reduce cardiac activity	Angina, hypertension, arrhythmia
Digoxin	Na^+/K^+-ATPase	Inhibitor	Positive inotropic activity	CHF
Dobutamine	β_1-Adrenoceptors	Agonist	Positive inotropic activity	CHF (acute)
Thiazide diuretic	Na^+/Cl^- transporter	Inhibitor	Promotes fluid loss	CHF
Loop diuretic	$Na^+/K^+/2Cl^-$ transporter	Inhibitor	Promotes fluid loss	CHF
ACE inhibitor (captopril)	Angiotensin-converting enzyme	Inhibitor	Prevents formation of angiotensin II	CHF, hypertension
Clonidine	α_2-Adrenoceptors	Agonist	Presynaptic inhibition of norepinephrine release (CNS)	Hypertension
Losartan	Angiotensin II receptor	Antagonist	Inhibits vasoconstriction, sympathetic stimulation, aldosterone synthesis and salt/water retention	Hypertension
Dihydropyridines	L-type calcium channel	Inhibitor	Reduce SA node activity (verapamil) and/or promote vasodilatation (nifedipine)	Hypertension
Prazosin	α_1-Adrenoceptors	Inhibitor	Interferes with sympathetic neurotransmission (indirect vasodilatation)	Hypertension
Minoxidil	K^+ (ATP) channels	Opener	Vasodilatation	Hypertension (severe)
Hydralazine	Guanylyl cyclase	Activator	Vasodilatation	Hypertension (severe, acute)
Sodium nitroprusside	Guanylyl cyclase (NO donor)	Activator	Vasodilatation	Hypertension (severe, emergency)
Haematinic drugs				
Aspirin	COX	Inhibitor	Prevents the formation of platelet thromboxane A_2 and reduces platelet aggregation	Prevention of embolic stroke, prevention of myocardial infarction in susceptible individuals

Continued

Table 1.3 EXAMPLES OF DRUGS THAT AFFECT BODY ORGANS—Cont'd

Agent/drug	Molecular target	Effect on target	Clinical effect	Condition
Clopidogrel	ADP receptor	Antagonist	Prevents platelet aggregation to ADP	As aspirin
Abciximab, tirofiban	Glycoprotein IIb/IIIa receptor	Antagonist	Prevent fibrinogen binding to platelets	Acute coronary syndromes
Heparin	Antithrombin III	Activates antithrombin III	Neutralizes clotting factors (Xa, IXa and thrombin)	Venous thromboembolism
Warfarin	Vitamin K reductase	Inhibitor	Inhibits synthesis of vitamin K-dependent clotting factors (II, VII, IX and X)	Venous and arterial thromboembolism
Streptokinase, alteplase (human recombinant tPA)	Plasminogen	Conversion to plasmin	Promote thrombus dissolution	Acute myocardial infarction, acute thrombotic stroke
Ferrous sulfate	Haemoglobin	Complex with haem	Required for synthesis of haemoglobin	Anaemia
Folic acid	Thymidylate synthase	Methyl donor	Synthesis of purines and pyrimidines	Anaemia
Vitamin B_{12}	Homocysteine–methionine methyltransferase	Cofactor	Synthesis of purines and pyrimidines	Anaemia
Desferrioxamine	Ferric ion	Chelation	Reduces iron overload	Thalassaemia major
Anti-inflammatory drugs				
Aspirin, ibuprofen	COX	COX1 selective inhibitor	Inhibit the production of prostaglandins	Analgesic, anti-inflammatory (rheumatoid arthritis, osteoarthritis), anti-pyretic
Fexofenadine	Histamine H_1 receptor	Antagonist	Inhibits histamine action	Allergic rhinitis, urticaria, drug hypersensitivities
Allopurinol	Xanthine oxidase	Inhibitor	Prevents the formation of uric acid	Gout
Probenecid	Organic anion transport (renal tubules)	Inhibitor	Promotes excretion of uric acid	Gout
Colchicine	Tubulin	Promotes microtubule depolymerization	Prevents neutrophil recruitment to the joint	Gout
Sulfasalazine	Inflammatory cells	Mechanism of action unclear	Inhibits inflammatory joint damage	Rheumatoid arthritis
Auranofin (gold compounds)	Inflammatory cells	Inhibits cytokine production	Inhibits inflammatory joint damage	Rheumatoid arthritis
Penicillamine	Inflammatory cells	Mechanism of action unclear	Inhibits inflammatory joint damage	Rheumatoid arthritis
Methotrexate	Dihydrofolate reductase	Inhibitor	Immunosuppressant	Rheumatoid arthritis
Azathioprine	DNA	Purine analogue	Inhibits DNA synthesis (e.g. immune cells)	Rheumatoid arthritis
Leflunomide	Dihydroorotate dehydrogenase	Inhibitor	Inhibits T cell function	Rheumatoid arthritis
Ciclosporin	Calcineurin	Inhibitor	Inhibits T cell function	Rheumatoid arthritis
Infliximab	TNFα	Antibody	Inhibits the actions of TNFα	Rheumatoid arthritis
Etanercept	TNFα	TNFα receptor	Inhibits the actions of TNFα	Rheumatoid arthritis
Anakinra	IL-1	Recombinant IL-1 receptor antagonist	Inhibits the actions of IL-1	Rheumatoid arthritis
Fluticasone propionate	Glucocorticosteroid receptor	Activation	Reduces inflammation	Asthma

COPD, chronic obstructive pulmonary disease; BPH, benign prostatic hyperplasia; SA, sinoatrial; AV, atrioventricular; CHF, chronic heart failure; COX, cyclooxygenase; TNF, tumour necrosis factor; IL-1, interleukin 1.

1 Drugs stimulate or inhibit biological processes by binding to specific proteins called receptors. Common receptor families include G-protein-coupled receptors, ion channels, receptor tyrosine kinases and intracellular receptors. Other proteins, such as enzymes and transporters, can also be targeted by drugs to alter their function.

2 An agonist mimics biological processes by binding to receptor, a process that depends on its affinity and ability to induce a conformational change (efficacy) in the receptor. Antagonists prevent agonists from binding to the receptor and inducing a conformational change in the protein. Antagonists must demonstrate affinity for a receptor but, unlike agonists, do not possess efficacy and can be described as competitive or irreversible competitive antagonists.

3 Drug absorption describes the process by which a drug enters the systemic circulation upon encountering a mucosal surface. The rate and extent of drug absorption is influenced by the physiochemical properties of the drug, including its size, shape, solubility at the site of absorption, degree of ionization and the relative lipid solubility of its non-ionized form. Distribution describes the process by which a drug enters the intercellular spaces surrounding tissue cells from the circulatory compartment and equilibrates with receptors on target cells. Drug distribution is influenced by plasma protein binding, solubility in adipose tissue, blood flow to tissues and membrane barriers.

4 The major site for drug biotransformation is the liver. Phase I biotransformations (e.g. oxidation) are catalysed by the cytochrome P450 (CYP) family of enzymes. The transformed species undergo a further conjugation reaction (phase II, e.g. glucuronidation) that terminates the biological activity of the parent molecule and promotes excretion by the kidney. The activity of the drug-metabolizing enzymes can be altered (e.g. by genetic variation or the presence of other drugs) and this has implications for clinical efficacy. In some cases, biotransformation can convert a prodrug into an active drug (e.g. conversion of codeine to morphine).

5 The parasympathetic nervous system is normally dominant during periods of inactivity (e.g. 'rest and digest') and promotes cardiac slowing, increased gastric motility and secretion. The sympathetic nervous system readies the body for physical exertion and promotes increased cardiac activity, increased blood flow to skeletal muscles, sweating, pupil dilation and mobilization of energy stores.

6 Acetylcholine is the parasympathetic nervous system neurotransmitter and rapidly activates muscarinic receptors on postjunctional membranes of effector cells to evoke a biological response. Muscarinic antagonists are a major drug class used to prevent the stimulatory actions of the parasympathetic nervous system and are used to treat motion sickness (hyoscine), in anaesthesia to prevent secretions and vagal slowing of the heart (hyosine), to prevent bronchoconstriction in asthma or chronic obstructive pulmonary disease (ipratropium bromide), in Parkinson's disease (benztropine), for gastric ulcers (pirenzipine) and for ophthalmological examination (tropicamide). Acetylcholinesterase inhibitors are used to augment cholinergic neurotransmission at the skeletal muscle junction in myasthenia gravis and to reverse the effects of competitive neuromuscular antagonists following surgery.

7 The activation of the sympathetic nervous system culminates in the release of norepinephrine from peripheral nerve endings and activation of adrenoceptors on effector cells. Many drugs interfere with sympathetic neurotransmission, including drugs that inhibit the enzymatic termination of norepinephrine (e.g. monamine oxidase inhibitors are used in the treatment of depression). Alpha-adrenoceptor agonists are used to promote vasoconstriction, which is a useful property for nasal decongestion (oxymetazoline) and retention of local anaesthetic at sites of injection. Beta-adrenoceptor stimulants are predominantly used in the treatment of respiratory diseases such as asthma and chronic obstructive pulmonary disease (salbutamol). Beta-blockers are widely used to prevent overstimulation of β-adrenoceptors in hypertension, arrhythmias, angina pectoris, glaucoma and anxiety.

8 Muscle paralysis may be desirable during surgery and can be induced by competitive antagonists of the skeletal muscle nicotinic receptor (e.g. rocuronium) or by non-depolarizing neuromuscular blockers (e.g. suxamethonium (succinylcholine)). In myasthenia gravis, antibodies directed against the end-plate nicotinic receptors impair motor coordination, and this can be treated with acetylcholinesterase inhibitors.

9 The opening of voltage-dependent sodium channels in nerve cells allows the entry of Na^+, membrane depolarization and spreading of an action potential along the length of the nerve. Local anaesthetics are weak bases that inactivate sodium channels, thereby reducing nerve excitability and impairing nerve conduction. These drugs are used in the treatment of pain (lidocaine, bupivacaine) and arrhythmias (lidocaine, mexiletine).

10 Arrhythmias are abnormal or irregular impulses by the heart and can lead to inefficient emptying of the ventricles, which may be life threatening. Treatment involves reducing the excitability of cardiac neuronal cells, thus allowing normal pacemaker rhythm to predominate. Four drug classes used in the treatment of arrhythmias inhibit sodium channels (class I, e.g. lidocaine), reduce sympathomimetic stimulation to the heart (class II, e.g. propranolol), inhibit potassium channels (class III, e.g. amiodarone) and inhibit calcium channels (class IV, verapamil).

11 Ischaemia of cardiac muscle manifests as a radiating chest pain when myocardial oxygen demand exceeds supply. Drugs used in the management of angina pectoris reduce preload to the heart (nitrovasodilators), cardiac contractility (beta-blockers), afterload (calcium channel blockers) and reduce the incidence of coronary thrombosis (aspirin).

12 A decrease in cardiac output because of a failing ventricle is characteristic of congestive heart failure and gives rise to symptoms of fatigue, fluid retention and difficulty in breathing (dyspnoea). Cardiac output can be improved with positive inotropic drugs (cardiac glycosides,

phosphodiesterase 3 inhibitors, β_1-agonists) and by reducing preload and congestion (diuretics, angiotensin-converting enzyme inhibitors, nitrovasodilators). The long-term use of beta-blockers appears to be beneficial in the treatment of this condition.

13 Hypertension is characterized by high blood pressure, usually of unknown aetiology although known risk factors include obesity, smoking, diabetes mellitus and hyperlipidaemia. A number of drug classes provide clinical benefit, including diuretic drugs (thiazides), which promote Na^+ and water loss and reduce vasoreactivity; drugs that interfere with the renin–angiotensin system, resulting in decreased total peripheral resistance and fluid loss (angiotensin-converting enzyme inhibitors, angiotensin II receptor antagonists); and drugs that reduce total peripheral resistance by promoting relaxation of peripheral resistance vessels (calcium channel blockers).

14 Activation of platelets and the coagulation cascade is critical for haemostasis. Under various pathological situations, thromboembolic events can be prevented by drugs that inhibit coagulation (heparin, warfarin), platelet aggregation (aspirin, ADP antagonists, GPIIb/IIIa antagonists and dipyramidol) and those that promote fibrinolysis (streptokinase, alteplase (tissue plasmin activator)).

15 Excess cholesterol in blood in the form of low density lipoprotein (LDL) promotes atherogenesis. A number of lipid-lowering drugs interfere with the absorption of cholesterol from the gastrointestinal tract (bile acid-binding resins), inhibit the synthesis of cholesterol and facilitate LDL clearance from the plasma (statins), inhibit extrahepatic lipase and promote clearance of VLDL (fibrates), inhibit the activity of hormone-sensitive lipase (nicotinic acid) and reduce the oxidant potential of LDL (probucol).

16 Red blood cell formation requires a number of important cofactors including iron, vitamin B_{12} and folic acid. A deficiency in the levels of these cofactors can lead to hypoproliferative anaemias characterized by microcytosis (iron deficiency) and macrocytosis (vitamin B_{12} and folate deficiency). Vitamin B_{12} is an important cofactor for the recycling of folate in cells and provides a biochemical link between B_{12} and folic acid metabolism. Supplementation with these cofactors can correct anaemia.

17 The kidney plays an important role in regulating body mineral and water content and a number of conditions, including nephrotic syndrome, liver disease and congestive heart failure, give rise to an accumulation of excessive fluid. Diuretics promote Na^+ excretion and water loss by a selective action in the kidney. These agents are also used in the treatment of hypertension. Diuretics include carbonic anhydrase inhibitors (acetazolamide), osmotic diuretics (mannitol), loop diuretics (furosemide), thiazide diuretics (indapamide) and potassium-sparing diuretics (amiloride, spironolactone).

18 Peptic ulcers are a result of imbalance between gastric acid secretion and secretion of cytoprotective factors. Pharmacological treatment involves reducing gastric acid production with proton pump inhibitors (omeprazole) and histamine H_2 receptor antagonists (cimetidine). Other agents promote cytoprotection (prostaglandins, sucralfate, bismuth chelate) and antibiotics eradicate *Helicobacter pylori* infection, a predisposing factor for peptic ulcers. Antacids (calcium carbonate) neutralize acid and have a beneficial action in the immediate relief of dyspepsia and gastro-oesophageal reflux.

19 Any change in gastrointestinal motility and secretion can significantly alter the transit of digested food in the gastrointestinal tract. In constipation, transit of digested foods may be increased with the aid of laxatives, including bulking agents, which stimulate motility (bran); salts (Epsom salts) and osmotic agents (lactulose) to increase bulk mass; stimulant laxatives (senna), which increase muscle motility; and faecal softeners (docusate). In diarrhoea, rehydration with fluid and electrolytes and the use of non-sedative opioids (loperamide) reduce transit time and facilitate absorption.

20 Nausea and emesis can occur postoperatively, during cancer therapy, following administration of drugs (contraceptives, non-steroidal anti-inflammatory drugs, opiates, dopamine) and through sensory stimuli (e.g. visual). Useful anti-emetic drugs such as $5HT_3$ receptor antagonists (ondansetron), dopamine D_2 receptor antagonists (metoclopramide, haloperidol), antihistamines (diphenhydramine), muscarinic antagonists (hyoscine), phenothiazines (chlorpromazine) and an NK_1 receptor antagonist (aprepitant) block activation of these receptors on neurons within the chemoreceptor trigger zone and vomiting centre.

21 Asthma is a disease of the airways characterized by reversible airway obstruction, inflammation of the resistance airways and bronchial hyperresponsiveness. Acute exacerbation of asthma can be controlled with bronchodilator drugs, of which several classes exist including β_2-adrenoceptor agonists (salbutamol) and anticholinergic drugs (ipratropium bromide). The underlying disease process can be controlled in part with glucocorticosteroids (budesonide), anti-allergic agents (disodium cromoglicate), xanthines (theophylline) and the cysteinyl-leukotriene antagonist (montelukast).

22 Chronic obstructive pulmonary disease (COPD) is a disease of the airways characterized by poorly reversible airway obstruction, inflammation of the resistance airways and destruction of alveoli. Bronchodilation is accomplished with bronchodilator drugs (β_2-adrenoceptor agonists, anticholinergic drugs). Apart from smoking cessation, there is currently no drug that modifies the underlying disease process. Glucocorticosteroids may be of some benefit in severe COPD.

23 Rhinitis is a common and debilitating disease characterized by rhinorrhoea (watery secretion), sneezing, itching, nasal congestion and obstruction; it may have allergic or non-allergic aetiology. Symptomatic treatment involves nasal decongestants (pseudoephedrine), antihistamines (cetirizine) and anticholinergic drugs (ipratropium bromide). Prophylactic treatment to suppress the underlying disease process utilizes glucocorticosteroids (beclomethasone diproprionate) and anti-allergic drugs (disodium cromoglicate). Newer agents include cysteinyl-leukotriene antagonists (montelukast) and biological agents such as the monoclonal IgE antibody (omalizumab).

24 Thyroid dysfunction is a common endocrinological problem. Excessive thyroid hormone production results in symptoms including tremor, palpitation and protruding eyes (Graves' disease). Anti-thyroid drugs like the thioureylenes (carbimazole) inhibit thyroid peroxidase and the synthesis and storage of thyroid hormone is impaired. Beta-blockers are used to treat the symptoms associated with overstimulation of the sympathetic nervous system. Radiolabelled iodine or thyroidectomy can be used to inhibit thyroid hormone production permanently in the case of carcinoma. Impaired thyroid hormone production (Hashimoto's thyroiditis) is associated with lethargy and cold intolerance; lifelong impairment can lead to loss in cognitive function and cretinism. Supplementation with thyroxine (levothyroxine, liothyronine) is required.

25 Type I diabetes is an autoimmune disease resulting in the destruction of pancreatic beta cells; as a result, subcutaneous injection of insulin following a meal is needed to stimulate glucose uptake into peripheral tissue. In type II diabetes, pancreatic beta cell function is impaired but insulin secretion can be stimulated by sulphonylureas (glipizide, glicazide) and non-sulphonylurea secretagogues (rapaglinide, nateglinide), and the increased peripheral resistance to the glucose uptake-promoting action of insulin can be reversed with biguanides (metformin) and glitazones (rosiglitazone, pioglitazone).

26 Corticosteroids synthesized in the adrenal cortex regulate carbohydrate, lipid and protein metabolism (cortisol) and electrolyte balance (aldosterone). In certain circumstances, the synthesis and release of corticosteroids may be impaired (Addison's disease) and this is treated with replacement therapy. In excessive glucocorticosteroid synthesis (Cushing's syndrome), surgery or treatment with drugs that impair the synthesis of glucocorticosteroids can be employed (aminoglutethimide). Glucocorticosteroids are also used utilized to treat inflammatory conditions (allergy, asthma, rheumatoid arthritis).

27 Oestrogen and progesterone are produced by the ovaries, regulate ovulation and prepare the female reproductive organ for implantation. This process can be inhibited with oral contraceptives, which suppress the hypothalamic–pituitary–adrenal axis thereby reducing gonadotrophin release and preventing ovulation. Hormone replacement therapy is often required in postmenopausal women and usually involves the administration of oestrogen with medroxyprogesterone in order to prevent symptoms of osteoporosis, hot flushes, vaginitis and increased low density lipoprotein cholesterol. Anti-oestrogens (tamoxifen) and aromatase inhibitors (anastrazole) are used in the treatment of breast cancer.

28 Testosterone and its more active metabolite dihydrotestosterone play an important role in male sexual development. Androgens are used clinically in the treatment of hypogonadism in males but can induce mascularization in women, and synthetic androgens have gained notoriety as performance-enhancing drugs. Androgen inhibitors, including receptor antagonists (flutamide) and inhibitors of 5α-reductase (finasteride), which is responsible for the conversion of testosterone to dihydrotestosterone, are used in the treatment of acne, hirsutism in women and in benign prostatic cancer.

29 Prostaglandins play a role in fever, thrombosis, pain and inflammation and are synthesized by cyclo-oxygenase (COX) in target cells. Aspirin irreversibly acetylates COX, which is of advantage in the management of thrombosis since platelet function can be selectively inhibited (as platelets contain no nucleus and so cannot regenerate enzyme). A variety of competitive non-steroidal anti-inflammatory agents (NSAIDs, e.g. diclofenac, naproxen, ibuprofen) with differing structure, potency and duration of action inhibit prostaglandin synthesis and are used in the treatment of fever, pain and inflammation. The major side-effect associated with NSAIDs is gastrointestinal bleeding, resulting from inhibition of the synthesis and action of 'protective' prostaglandins.

30 Overstimulation of the body's immune system leads to rheumatoid arthritis, a chronic inflammatory condition associated with joint erosion, inflammation, swelling and pain. Immunosuppressant drugs (ciclosporin) and disease-modifying drugs (DMARDS; methotrexate) inhibit immune cell function and treat the underlying inflammation. NSAIDs treat the symptoms of pain but do not modify the underlying inflammatory condition. Newer biological agents target cytokines such as tumour necrosis factor (infliximab, etanercept) and interleukin 1 (anakinra) that are implicated in the disease process.

31 Urinary incontinence is a consequence of over-activity of the bladder (UUI) or inability to retain urine (SSI). UUI is treated with antimuscarinic agonists (tolterodine, darifenacin), which impair the excitatory actions of the parasympathetic nervous system; SSI is treated by increasing urethral smooth muscle activity with α-adrenoceptor agonists (midodrine, phenylpropanolamine) or by inhibiting the urge to void using centrally acting drugs (duloxetine). Urethral obstruction can result from enlargement of the prostate, which can occur in benign prostatic hyperplasia or prostatic cancer. Gland size can be reduced by the use of non-selective α_1-adrenoceptor antagonists (tamsulosin, doxazosin), which induce relaxation of the urethral smooth muscle, and 5α-reductase inhibitors (finasteride, dutasteride (α_1-antagonists), which reduce proliferation of prostatic epithelium. Male erectile dysfunction is an inability to develop and maintain an erection. Inhibitors of phosphodiesterase 5 (sildenafil) promote an erection by preventing the inactivation of cGMP within cavernosal smooth muscle cells, which promotes increased blood flow and tumescence. Intracavernosal injection of alprostadil raises intracellular levels of cAMP, which also increases blood flow and hence an erection. Uterine motility can be stimulated with oxytocin. Premature labour can be suppressed by tocolytic agents that inhibit uterine contraction, including β-adrenoceptor agonists (terbutaline, ritodrine), magnesium sulphate and calcium channel blockers (nifedipine).

32 Overproduction or impaired drainage of aqueous humour within the anterior chamber of the eye leads to increased intraocular pressure and glaucoma. The production of aqueous humour by the ciliary body can be inhibited by beta-blockers (timolol), carbonic anhydrase inhibitors (dorzolamide) and α_2-adrenoceptor agonists (apraclonidine, brimonidine). Intraocular pressure can also be relieved by increasing the outflow of aqueous humour using muscarinic agonists (pilocarpine) and prostaglandins (latanoprost).

33 A number of conditions affecting the skin (acne, psoriasis and dermatitis) are amenable to pharmacological treatment. Acne is caused by excessive sebum production and infection with bacteria and it can be treated with benzoyl peroxide and, in severe cases, with antibiotics. Excessive proliferation of keratinocytes, which help to trap sebum within the sebaceous follicle unit, can be inhibited with salicylic acid, azelaic acid and topical retinoids (tazarotene). Psoriasis is characterized by rapid proliferation of the epidermis, resulting in scaling erythematous plaques, which can be treated with tars, phototherapy (ultraviolet B plus psoralens), vitamin D analogues (calcipotriene, tacalcitol) and topical retinoids (tazarotene). Dermatitis is characterized by uncontrolled scratching and inflammation of the dermis and is treated with anti-inflammatory agents (glucocorticosteroids), immunosuppressants (ciclosporin) and cytotoxic drugs (azathioprine, methotrexate). Antihistamines (cetirizine) have some clinical benefit.

34 Parkinson's disease is a movement disorder resulting from loss of substantia nigral dopaminergic neurons innervating the striatum and control of thalamic neuron activity to the motor cortex. This disruption in neural activity results in slow (bradykinesia) and rigid movement, resting tremor and disturbances in gait. Treatment involves the supplementation with levodopa, which significantly improves symptoms but requires functioning dopaminergic neurons innervating the striatum. Prolonged treatment with levodopa results in dyskinesia (impaired movement); this unwanted side-effect can be delayed by initiating treatment with dopamine-selective agonists (bromocriptine). Other treatments include preventing the metabolism of dopamine with monoamine oxidase B inhibitors (selegiline) and catechol-O-methyl-transferase inhibitors (entacapone). Anticholinergic drugs (trihexyphenidyl) and the antiviral agent amantadine are also used.

35 Drugs used in the treatment of anxiety include benzodiazepines, which reduce neuronal excitability by facilitating the opening of GABA$_A$ receptors and Cl$^-$ entry into postsynaptic neurons. They provide rapid anxiolytic action although they suffer from occurrence of withdrawal symptoms (rebound anxiety) and drug dependence. Non-benzodiazepine drugs, zopiclone, zolpidem and zaleplon, are short-acting hypnotic agents that have higher affinity for the benzodiazepine-binding site and, therefore, have reduced potential for drug dependence and withdrawal symptoms. A number of other drugs used in the treatment of some forms of anxiety include agents that target serotonergic neurotransmission, including buspirone (5HT$_{1A}$-receptor agonist), the serotonin selective reuptake inhibitors (SSRI; fluoxetine, paroxetine, sertraline), the monamine oxidase inhibitors (moclobemide) and the tricyclic antidepressants (imipramine, doxepine). Beta-blockers can also be used to reduce the peripheral action of overstimulation of the sympathetic nervous system during anxiety.

36 Depression is thought to be caused by impaired norepinephrine and serotonergic activity in the CNS. The tricyclic antidepressants (imipramine, doxepin) inhibit the uptake of biogenic amines into nerve terminals and the monamine oxidase inhibitors (moclobemide) inhibit their metabolism, thereby increasing the levels of these amines at synapses between neurons. Newer more tolerable antidepressants include serotonin selective reuptake inhibitors (fluoxetine, paroxetine), selective norepinephrine/serotonin reuptake inhibitors (venla-faxine, duloxetine) and the norepinephrine reuptake inhibitor roboxetine. Other agents include mirtazapine (α_2-adrenoceptor and 5HT$_{2A,3}$ receptor antagonist), bupro-pion (norepinephrine reuptake inhibitor, 5HT$_{1A}$ receptor agonist) and the atypical antidepressants trazodone and nefazodone (serotonin reuptake inhibitor, 5HT$_{2A}$ receptor antagonist). Mood stabilizers include lithium and a number of neuroleptic drugs, such as sodium valproate and carbamazepine.

37 The clinical efficacy of antipsychotic drugs correlates with their affinity for dopamine D$_2$ receptors. Haloperidol is an example of this drug class but the group of drugs suffers from extrapyramidal side-effects caused by blockade of D$_2$ receptors in the striatum. Atypical antipsychotic drugs (e.g. clozapine) have lower affinity for striatal D$_2$ receptors than typical antipsychotic drugs and, therefore, are free from extrapyramidal side-effects. They show higher affinity for serotonin than dopamine receptors and highlight an important role for serotonergic neurons in schizophrenia.

38 Epilepsy is characterized by seizures and can be broadly classified as generalized (both hemispheres) or partial (localized) syndromes. The molecular basis of epilepsies involves neuronal hyperexcitability, and drug therapy is achieved by enhancing GABAergic activity (barbiturates, benzodiazepines) and inhibiting sodium (phenytoin, carbamazepine, sodium valproate) and calcium (ethosuximide) channels. Sodium valproate has additional properties that account for its antiseizure activity, including enhancing GABAergic neuron activity and blocking T-type calcium channels. Drugs such as ethosuximide and sodium valproate are useful in absence seizures. Established anti-epileptic drugs induce P450 CYP activity and, therefore, interfere with the metabolism of other drugs.

39 General anaesthesia is induced with intravenous anaesthetics, thiopental (barbiturate), propofol, etomidate and ketamine (non-barbiturate). Maintenance anaesthesia is usually performed with a gaseous anaes-thetic (nitrous oxide, isoflurane, enflurane, sevoflurane). Other agents may also be administered as premedication including opiates (analgesia), antimuscarinic agents (reduce secretions) and benzodiazepines (reduce anxiety). Neuromuscular-blocking agents may also be employed in surgical procedures.

40 A number of drug classes are used to reduce the symptoms of a migraine attack and include NSAIDs, ergot derivatives and triptans (sumitriptan). The triptans are selective agonists for serotonin $5HT_{1B/1D/1F}$ receptors and promote cerebral vessel vasoconstriction, inhibit neurotransmitter release and activation of pain-sensing nerves. Because of their vasoconstrictor properties, they should not be used in patients with ischaemic heart disease, hypertension and cerebrovascular disease. A number of pharmacological agents are also used prophylactically in an attempt to prevent the onset of migraine and include beta-blockers, anticonvulsants (sodium valproate) and antidepressants (amitriptyline, nortriptyline).

41 Endogenous opioids regulate pain transmission by activating G-protein-coupled receptors present on spinal and supraspinal nerves. The opioid μ-receptor subtypes mediate most of the analgesic actions of opioids (morphine, codeine). Opioids can also be used for the treatment of cough (dextromethorphan) and as anti-diarrhoeal agents (loperamide). Chronic use of opiates can lead to tolerance and to psychological and physical dependence. Methadone is used because of its long half-life to treat drug addiction by reducing the intensity of the withdrawal symptoms.

42 A variety of substances can give rise to drug dependence, which is associated with an intense desire or craving for the drug and the development of tolerance with continued use (higher concentrations of the drug needed to satisfy the addiction). Opiates, CNS stimulants (amphetamines, cocaine), CNS depressants (ethanol, benzodiazepines), cannabinoids and nicotine give rise to drug dependence. The interaction of these substances with dopaminergic pathways in the CNS is thought to play a major role in drug dependence.

43 Antimicrobial activity can be achieved by disrupting the peptidoglycan layer of bacterial wall with β-lactams such as the penicillins (flucloxacillin), cephalosporins (cefotaxime), carbapenems (meropenem) and monobactams (aztreonam). Resistance can develop through occurrence of a bacterial β-lactamase but this can be negated by inhibitors (clavulanate), which, therefore, prolong the activity of non-enzyme-resistant β-lactams. The glycopeptides (vancomycin) also target the formation of peptidoglycans, but at a different step to the β-lactams, and have been very useful in treating β-lactam-resistant strains (e.g. methicillin-resistant *Staphylococcus aureus*; MRSA). Other antimicrobial agents inhibit bacterial

nucleic acid synthesis: the antifolates sulphonamides and trimethoprim inhibit production of the building units for nucleic acid synthesis; the fluroquinolones (ciprofloxacin) inhibit DNA unwinding via action on bacterial DNA gyrase (topoisomerase II); and the rifamycins (rifampin) bind to bacterial RNA polymerase.

44 Agents affecting bacterial protein synthesis are bacteriostatic, with the exception of aminoglycosides and oxazolidinones. Tetracyclines and aminoglycosides interfere with protein synthesis by binding to the 30S ribosomal subunit. Among the aminoglycosides, gentamicin is most commonly used to treat infections by Gram-negative bacteria, tobramycin is used for *Pseudomonas aeruginosa* and streptomycin for *Mycobacterium tuberculosis*. The side-effects of this drug class limit its utility. The macrolides and lincosamides bind to the 50S ribosomal subunit and are active against Gram-positive bacteria. The streptogramins prevent elongation of the peptide chain. Two streptogramins, quinupristin and dalfopristin, combined (3:7, respectively) are very effective against infections with staphylococci, streptococci and against vancomycin-resistant *Enterococcus faecalis* and methicillin-resistant *Staphylococcus aureus*. They are used against catheter-related infections, endocarditis, bacteraemia and soft-tissue infections.

45 Antiviral agents target viral entry (amantadine) and exit (neuraminidase inhibitors), DNA replication and protein synthesis. Immunoglobulins specific for antigenic determinants on cell surface viral protein can bind and neutralize the ability of virus to infect host cells and improve clearance of the virus from the host (e.g. anti-hepatitis B). For DNA viruses, DNA replication is prevented by agents that in their triphosphate active forms (aciclovir) can inhibit DNA polymerase. Other inhibitors of viral DNA synthesis include phosphonoformates (foscarnet) and nucleoside analogues (tribavarin).

46 Retroviruses on entering a host cell use reverse transcriptase to synthesize DNA from viral RNA and this enzyme can be inhibited by nucleoside reverse transcriptase inhibitors (zidovudine) and non-nucleoside reverse transcriptase inhibitors (nevirapine, efavirenz). Protease inhibitors (saquinavir) inhibit the synthesis of viral proteins and do not require phosphorylation to become active. The human immunodeficiency virus (HIV) is a retrovirus that is presently causing a pandemic; it destroys the cells of the immune system, leading to the acquired immunodeficiency syndrome (AIDS) and death. Because HIV mutates rapidly, resistance develops quite easily to many of the drugs used in its treatment. As a result, drugs are combined into complex regimens of three or more drugs, known as highly active antiretroviral therapy (HAART).

47 An effective anthelmintic must penetrate the cuticle of the worm or gain access to its alimentary tract. Drugs can act by causing paralysis of the worm or by damaging its cuticle, which can alert the host immune defences to remove the parasite, or by interfering with its metabolism. The last group tends to be very specific for a particular type of worm. The benzimidazoles (e.g. thiabendazole) inhibit glucose uptake in the parasite and inhibit the polymerization and breakdown of cytoskeleton microtubules. Praziquantel, an effective broad-spectrum anthelmintic against trematodes and cestodes, appears to interfere with Ca^{2+} homeostasis, resulting in paralysis and detachment of the helminth. Ivermectin prevents closure of GABA-ergic chloride-sensitive channels, leading to tonic paralysis of the nematode's muscle system and death.

48 Malaria is a parasitic infection transmitted by the *Anopheles* mosquito, which carries sporozoites of the *Plasmodium* spp. that infect the human host. A number of drug classes target different stages of the protozoal life cycle in the mammalian host. Drugs structurally derived from quinine (chloroquine) and derivatives of arteminsin (artesunate) target the red blood cell stage and interfere with the ability of these protozoa to detoxify free haem and digest haemoglobin. Arteminsin derivatives work much faster than conventional anti-malarial drugs and when used in combination regimens (artesunate and mefloquine) reduce the risk of the development of resistance. Type I (sulphonamides) and type II (pyrimethamine) antifolates prevent protozoal DNA transcription. Primaquine targets the tissue stage of these protozoa by inhibiting DNA and mitochondrial respiration.

49 A number of drug classes used against fungal infection target the fungal envelope (wall and membrane). The structural integrity of this envelope can be compromised by drugs that either bind to ergosterol, an important structural protein of fungal envelope (polyene macrolides: amphotericin B, nystatin) or inhibit its synthesis (at distinct sites along the biosynthetic pathway, e.g. ketoconazole, terbinafine, amorolfine). Capsofungin targets the synthesis of another constituent of the fungal envelope ($\beta(1,3)$-glycans). Drugs that target microtubule assembly (griseofulvin) and DNA synthesis (flucytosine) also show antifungal activity.

50 Malignant tumours can be treated by drugs that directly alkylate DNA (cyclophosphamide), promote DNA strand breaks and hence cell cycle arrest by inter-calation with DNA (antitumour antibiotics; doxorubicin) or prevent DNA resealing by inhibiting topoisomerase II (irinotecam). Some agents act earlier by interfering with the synthesis of nucleoside building blocks, for example the antifolates (methotrexate), pyrimidine analogues (5-flurouracil) and purine analogues (mercaptopurine). The disruption of microtubule formation will also disrupt cell proliferation and this is achieved with agents that inhibit (vinca alkaloids; vinblastine) or promote (paclitaxel) polymerization of microtubules. Hormonal or antihormonal therapy is used in the treatment of breast (tamoxifen, anastrozole) or prostate (flutamide) cancer. More recently, antibodies and small molecule inhibitors targeting growth-promoting proteins have been developed. Hence, antibodies have been used to target haematological neoplasms (rituximab in B cell lymphoma) and solid tumours (trastuzumab in breast cancer). Small molecule inhibitors have been developed for the treatment of myeloid leukaemia (imatinib mesylate) and non-small cell lung cancer (gefitinib).

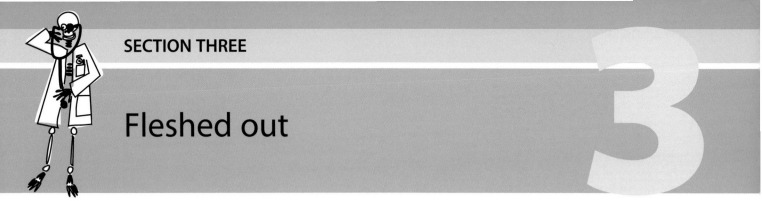

SECTION THREE

Fleshed out

Section 3 builds on the information covered in The big picture and each chapter covers in a little more detail the pharmacology of drug action. In the first two chapters, the nature of drugs and their interaction with drug targets are defined. The body has evolved systems to metabolize and excrete chemicals and it is, therefore, an important determinant of how a drug will act, which is the subject of the next two chapters. Chapters 5–9 highlight the mechanisms by which neurotransmitters alter cell function and the potential targets for drug action at the interface between the autonomic nervous system and neuroeffector cells. The following chapters describe the pharmacology of important drugs used in the cardiovascular system (Chs 10–14, 16), liver (Ch. 15), kidney (Ch. 17), gastrointestinal tract (Chs 18–20), respiratory system (Chs 21–23), endocrine glands (Chs 24–26), reproductive tract (Chs 27 and 28); urinogenitory tract (Ch. 31), eye (Ch. 32), skin (Ch. 33) and central nervous system (Chs 34–42). Drugs that target inflammatory processes are covered in Chapters 29 and 30 while drugs targeting pathogens are covered in Chapters 43–49 and cancer is covered in Chapter 50.

1. Principles of drug action

Questions
- How can a drug be defined?
- What are the types of receptor?

Under normal physiological conditions, hormones (e.g. epinephrine) or neurotransmitters (e.g. acetylcholine) play an important role in transmitting information from one cell to another. They do so by binding to and inducing an alteration in the conformational state (structure) of specific proteins (**receptors**).

Drugs
Drugs are chemicals that alter the biological response of cells. Their chemical structure often mimics a natural substance in the body but they can be chemically distinct; in either case they selectively target receptors (Fig. 3.1.1). The binding of a drug to its receptor is the first step in a series of complex reactions inside the cell that ultimately evokes a therapeutic effect and, therefore, provides a 'magic bullet' for the treatment of disease. The drug can either initiate an endogenous process or inhibit the action of endogenous hormones and neurotransmitters.

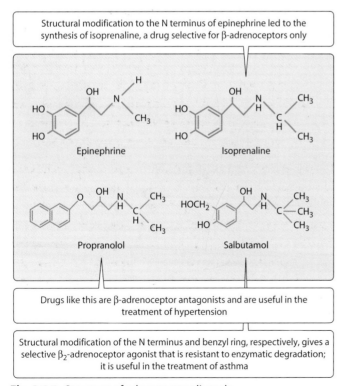

Structural modification to the N terminus of epinephrine led to the synthesis of isoprenaline, a drug selective for β-adrenoceptors only

Epinephrine   Isoprenaline

Propranolol   Salbutamol

Drugs like this are β-adrenoceptor antagonists and are useful in the treatment of hypertension

Structural modification of the N terminus and benzyl ring, respectively, gives a selective β₂-adrenoceptor agonist that is resistant to enzymatic degradation; it is useful in the treatment of asthma

Fig. 3.1.1 Structure of adrenoceptor ligands.

Receptors
There are many different types of receptor found on the surface or inside cells. Receptors within cells can be situated either in the cytoplasm or in the nucleus, bound to regions of DNA (response elements) near genes whose activity is to be regulated.

G-protein-coupled receptors. This large protein family comprises cell surface receptors (e.g. β-adrenoceptor, muscarinic receptor) that are activated by hormones and neurotransmitters. A characteristic feature of these receptors is that they contain seven membrane-spanning domains and their activation leads to the subsequent synthesis of intracellular second messengers, which activate numerous proteins within cells as an amplification cascade (Fig. 3.1.2).

Ion channels. Some cell surface proteins contain a pore domain (e.g. nicotinic receptor, calcium channel) that when opened allows the movement of ions down their concentration gradient. These channels can be either receptor operated (ROC) or voltage operated (VOC). Examples of ROCs include the nicotinic acetylcholinergic receptor. Voltage-gated ion channels are activated by alterations in cell membrane potential. The channel can sense the voltage of the surrounding membrane and becomes activated (i.e. opens) when the voltage is altered, leading to the influx or efflux of ions (e.g. Na^+, Ca^{2+} or K^+). Activation of a sodium or calcium channel in nerves results in nerve depolarization and neurotransmitter release, respectively. The activation of potassium channels in nerves leads to membrane hyperpolarization and inhibition of cell excitability.

Receptor tyrosine kinases. A characteristic feature of these receptors is that ligand binding (e.g. insulin and erythropoietin) to the receptor on the surface of the cell leads to the formation of receptor complexes (dimers and tetramers) and phosphorylation of tyrosine residues on numerous intracellular proteins. This triggers a cascade of events leading to cell activation (e.g. the platelet-derived growth factor initiates the proliferation of smooth muscle) (Fig. 3.1.3). These proteins are involved in the regulation of cell growth, differentiation and activity.

Intracellular receptors. These receptors are usually found within the cytoplasm (e.g. glucocorticosteroid) or bound to DNA (e.g. thyroid). Binding of the hormone to its receptor leads to the movement of the drug–receptor complex to specific sites near the promoter regions of genes, thereby modulating the rate of gene transcription (see Fig. 1.2D). For example, glucocorticosteroids promote expression of the anti-inflammatory protein lipocortin, which inhibits

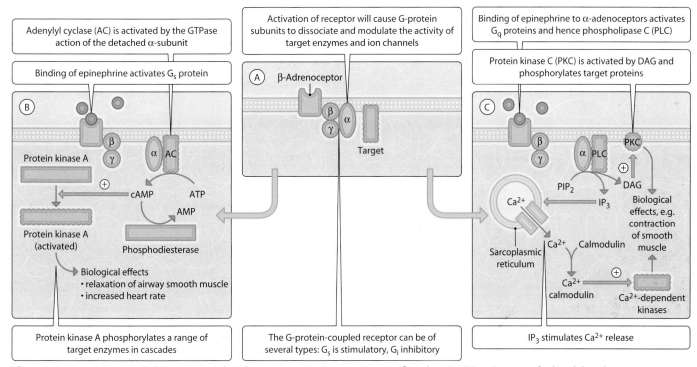

Fig. 3.1.2 G-protein-coupled receptors. (A) Linkage occurs to targets via specific subunits; (B) activation of adenylyl cyclase; (C) activation of phospholipase C. PIP$_2$, phosphatidylinositol 4,5-bisphosphate; IP$_3$, inositol 1,4,5-trisphosphate; DAG, diacylglycerol.

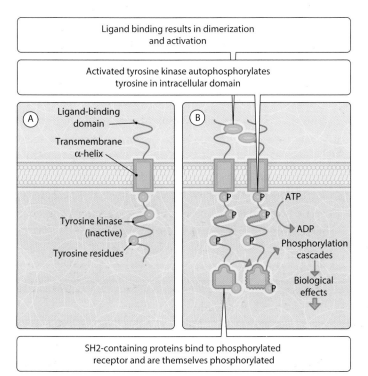

Fig. 3.1.3 Transduction by tyrosine kinase-linked receptors.

phospholipase A$_2$, an enzyme involved in the metabolism of arachidonic acid to prostaglandins and leukotrienes. These receptors are often involved in the control of growth, reproduction and cell homeostasis.

Other proteins. There is a diverse group of proteins (e.g. enzymes) that regulate the function of cells by catalysing the reaction of various molecules. Thus, acetylcholinesterase is a membrane-bound enzyme found on the surface of neurons and postjunctional effector sites. This enzyme hydrolyses acetylcholine, thereby terminating its pharmacological activity. The activity of this enzyme can be inhibited with an acetycholinesterase inhibitor (e.g. organophosphates).

The movement of ions and molecules across the cell membrane by transport/carrier proteins is an important requirement for cell homeostasis. Some of these pumps are energy dependent. A classical example is sodium/potassium adenosine triphosphatase (Na$^+$/K$^+$-ATPase). This protein pumps Na$^+$ from inside cells to the extracellular spaces and K$^+$ from outside cells to the inside in an energy-dependent process. These ions can then flow down their concentration gradient when the appropriate ion channel is opened.

2. Drug–receptor interactions

Questions
- What is drug affinity?
- What is drug efficacy?
- How do antagonists differ from agonists?

Agonists

The binding of a hormone, neurotransmitter or drug to its receptor is, in most cases, a reversible process that can be described by the law of mass action (Fig. 3.2.1). At equilibrium, the rates of drug–receptor complex association and dissociation are equal. The equilibrium is determined by the affinity of the drug for its receptor and by the drug and receptor concentrations. This can be examined in binding studies in which a drug labelled with a radioisotope is incubated with a homogenate of membranes from tissues or cells. Washing removes any unbound drug and the retained radioactivity (after correction for non-specific binding) most likely reflects binding to the receptor of interest.

A number of useful parameters are derived from this relationship (Fig. 3.2.1A). The concentration of drug required to occupy 50% of the total number of receptors available is denoted by K_D and is a measure of **drug affinity**. In general, drugs with high binding affinity have very low K_D values (i.e. nanomolar) and, therefore, would be advantageous for the treatment of diseases, since the drug would selectively bind to the desired target but not to other proteins, thus reducing side-effects.

Some agonists are better than others at eliciting a biological response because they are better able to induce a conformational change in the receptor protein (Fig. 3.2.1B). This transition to an activated complex is a prerequisite for a biological response. The ability of an agonist to induce a conformational change in the receptor is its **efficacy**. Drugs with high efficacy have a greater propensity to induce a conformational change in the receptor than drugs with low efficacy, producing maximum biological response while activating only a fraction of the available receptor pool. In most cases, such drugs are often referred to as full agonists. Agonists with low efficacy, and therefore less able to evoke the full biological response despite occupying all of the available receptors, are termed partial agonists. Note that partial or full agonists will also possess their own particular affinity for a receptor (Fig. 3.2.2). **Potency** describes the 'strength' of a drug and is evaluated as the EC_{50} (concentrate evoking 50% of maximum response). It is a useful measure of how good a drug is at evoking a response and is dependent on drug affinity and efficacy.

Antagonists

A drug that prevents the actions of an agonist is classified as an antagonist. An antagonist has affinity for a receptor but does not

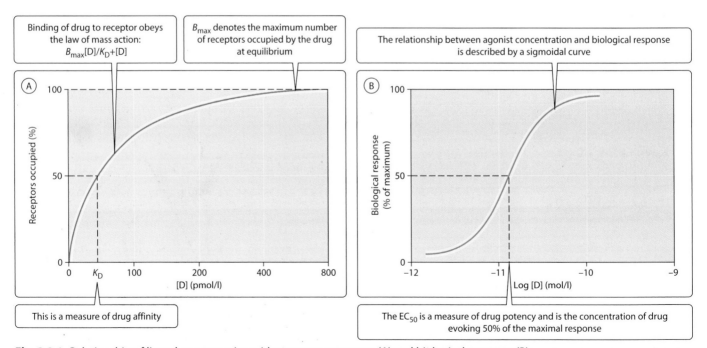

Fig. 3.2.1 Relationship of ligand concentration with receptor occupancy (A) and biological response (B).

produce a conformational change in the receptor protein. Under such circumstances, the chemical is said to have affinity for the receptor but no efficacy. There are two main classes of drug receptor antagonist: competitive and irreversible.

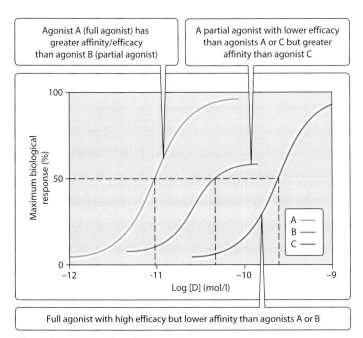

Fig. 3.2.2 Full and partial agonists.

A **competitive (reversible) antagonist** competes with the agonist for the same receptor (Fig. 3.2.3A; e.g. atropine (muscarinic receptor)). This antagonism can be overcome by increasing the concentration of the agonist. Experimentally, this can be seen as a rightward shift in the agonist concentration–response curve in the presence of increasing concentrations of antagonist. A linear plot of the logarithm of the dose ratio (i.e. ratio of agonist EC50 in the absence versus presence of antagonist) minus one against antagonist concentration yields a Schild plot, from which the affinity of the antagonist can be derived.

An **irreversible competitive antagonist** binds covalently to the agonist-binding site on the receptor (e.g. phenoxybenzamine binding to α-adrenoceptors). Agonist can compete with the antagonist before the covalent bond forms but once it has, the antagonism is insurmountable. This causes a downward shift in the concentration–response curve to the agonist (Fig. 3.2.3B).

A **non-competitive antagonist** can act at an allosteric site, ion channel or site distal to the receptor and non-specifically blocks the action of an agonist (eg calcium channel blocker prevents vasoconstriction).

Other forms of antagonism are **chemical**, where one drug binds another thereby inactiviting it (protamine with heparin), and **physiological**, where the action of one drug opposes the action of a second agent (salbutamol with acetylcholine).

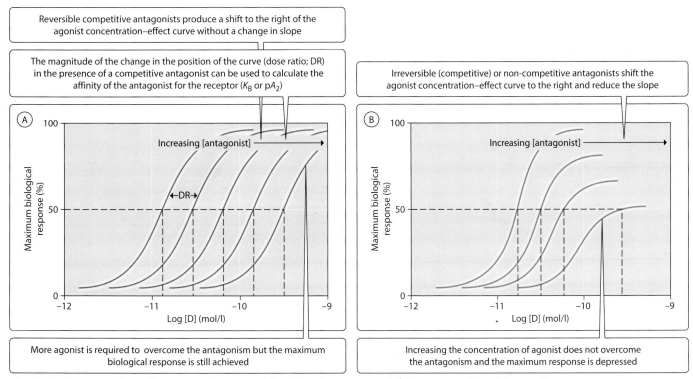

Fig. 3.2.3 Concentration–effect curves for competitive (A) and non-competitive (B) antagonists of drug action.

3. Pharmacokinetics: absorption and distribution

Questions
- What factors govern drug absorption?
- What routes can be used for dosing?
- What factors govern drug distribution?

Absorption

Drugs can be administered by a number of routes:

- **oral**: convenient but drugs are subject to first pass metabolism in the liver and it is not suitable for agents readily destroyed by bacterial enzymes or the acid environment of the stomach (e.g. insulin) unless the drug is protected in some way (e.g. a coated tablet). Drug absorption by this route is altered by gastric motility, pH at the site of absorption, mucosal blood flow and the presence of food
- **sublingual**: bypasses the problems affecting oral drugs (e.g. nitroglycerin)
- **inhalation**: suitable for general anaesthetics and when the lung is a target for therapy (e.g. salbutamol in asthma); it minimizes systemic levels of drug because a lower total dose can be given and any swallowed portion will be subject to first pass metabolism
- **subcutaneous (s.c.) or intramuscular (i.m.) (injection)**: useful for drugs in aqueous form; drugs can be formulated to slow the rate of absorption (e.g. contraceptive implants)
- **parenteral (intravenous (i.v.) injection)**: advantageous for rapid pharmacological effect and when continuous infusion is required

- **rectal (suppository)**: avoids first pass metabolism because there is limited portal blood flow from the lower gastro-intestinal tract.

In order for a drug to be absorbed into the systemic circulation, it must be able to cross cell membranes. These membranes are mainly composed of lipids so lipophilic molecules will readily diffuse across these structures. Most drugs exist in an ionized (charged) and a non-ionized (uncharged) form in solution and it is the latter that readily penetrate cell membranes. The amount of drug absorbed across cell membranes will depend upon the amount of drug in the non-ionized form (Fig. 3.3.1). The extent to which a drug is non-ionized will be dependent upon the pH of the environment and the drug's pK_A (negative logarithm of K_A). The pK_A is equal to the pH at which 50% of a drug is ionized in solution (Fig. 3.3.1). Some charged molecules can be transported across cell membranes by specific carrier proteins residing in the cell membrane.

Increasing gastric emptying can limit absorption of a drug from the stomach but will hasten the absorption of weak bases from the lower intestine. Slowing gastric emptying will tend to delay drug absorption from the small intestine. Following absorption from the gastrointestinal tract, drugs reach the liver via the portal circulation; if they are metabolized in the liver (**first pass metabolism**) this will prevent unchanged drug reaching the systemic circulation.

Distribution

In the simplest model, the body is considered a single uniform space (compartment) where drug enters and leaves (elimination) and it is assumed that the drug is immediately distributed throughout the body (Fig. 3.3.2). The elimination of drug obeys first-order kinetics and is proportional to the concentration of drug in the plasma. This can be represented mathematically as an exponential loss of drug from the body (Fig. 3.3.3). This loss reflects drug distributed throughout the body and elimination from the body. A number of useful parameters concerning a drugs distribution within the body can be obtained from this relationship.

Volume of distribution. The extent of distribution of the drug throughout the body compartment is referred to as the apparent volume of distribution (V_d). This is the theoretical volume into which a drug instantaneously equilibrates on entering the body compartment. It gives an indication of the amount of drug remaining in the blood but gives no indication as to where the drug has accumulated. A very high

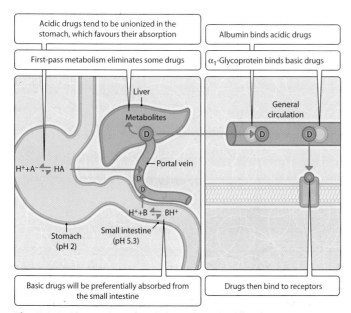

| Acidic drugs tend to be unionized in the stomach, which favours their absorption | Albumin binds acidic drugs |
| First-pass metabolism eliminates some drugs | α_1-Glycoprotein binds basic drugs |

Liver
Metabolites
General circulation
$H^+ + A^- \rightleftharpoons HA$
Portal vein
$H^+ + B \rightleftharpoons BH^+$
Stomach (pH 2)
Small intestine (pH 5.3)

| Basic drugs will be preferentially absorbed from the small intestine | Drugs then bind to receptors |

Fig. 3.3.1 Absorption of oral drugs into the bloodstream.

V_d value suggests that the drug is preferentially distributed throughout the body organs resulting in a low plasma concentration (e.g. distributed in adipose tissue or bound to proteins in body organs). Conversely, a drug that preferentially binds to plasma protein will be retained within the circulation and will be characterized by values of V_d approaching that of plasma volume. For many drugs, V_d may be considerably greater than the actual body weight and this is an indication that the drug has greater affinity for tissues than plasma.

Plasma half-life.   The elimination rate constant is a useful parameter describing how quickly a drug is eliminated from the blood compartment, but a more common term is the plasma half-life ($t_{1/2}$), which is the time for plasma drug concentrations to decline by 50%; because plasma drug concentration declines linearly over time, the half-life will be constant regardless of drug concentration (Fig. 3.3.3B,C). Knowing plasma half-life is important, particularly when drugs have to be administered over long periods of time.

A variety of factors can influence drug distribution throughout the body compartment.

- Drugs with high affinity for plasma protein will have limited access to tissue cells and their receptors but will be protected from elimination and so are retained in the body for a longer period. As the plasma concentration of drug falls owing to elimination and/or equilibration to organs, drug will dissociate from plasma protein.
- Drugs that are relatively lipid insoluble (or highly ionized) will have slower access across capillary membranes and will be eliminated relatively quickly, while lipid-soluble drugs will tend to accumulate to a greater extent in fat stores and will be eliminated more slowly from the body compartment.
- Drugs will distribute predominantly but rapidly to organs with the largest blood supply, including the heart, liver and kidney. Delivery to muscle, viscera, skin and fat is slower.
- Access to the cerebrospinal fluid and extracellular spaces of the brain are constrained by the blood–brain barrier (endothelial cells lining the capillaries in the brain); drugs that are extremely polar such as quaternary amines are unable to gain access to the CNS, although the barrier may become more permeable in disease. Some areas of the CNS are not behind this barrier (e.g. area postrema, involved in triggering nausea and vomiting to noxious substances).

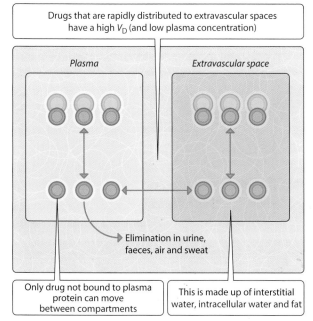

Fig. 3.3.2 Drug distribution.

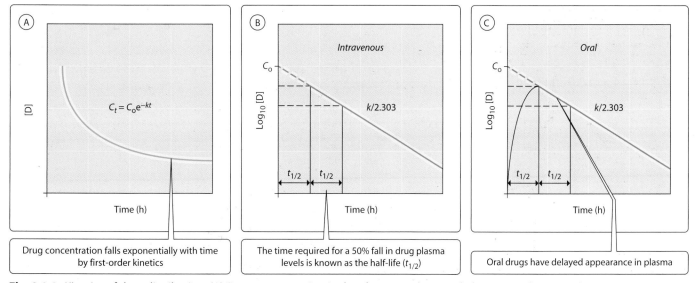

Fig. 3.3.3 Kinetics of drug distribution. (A) Drug concentration in the plasma can be sampled over time from initial concentration C_0. (B,C) Plotting as $\log_{10}$ gives a linear plot with a delay in drug appearance for oral administration.

4. Pharmacokinetics: metabolism and excretion

Questions
- How are drugs metabolized?
- How are drugs excreted?
- What factors alter drug excretion?

Drug metabolism

The liver is the major organ for the biotransformation of drugs. Hepatic cytochrome P450 (CYP) actively metabolizes endogenous and exogenous chemicals to metabolites that are, in general, more polar; this promotes elimination from the body and terminates drug action. In some cases, the metabolite may itself have potent biological activity or have toxic properties. Essentially, two types of biotransformation can occur.

Phase 1. CYP belongs to a family of haem-containing enzymes and is the major catalyst of drug biotransformation involving oxidative and reductive reactions. It has evolved to biotransform a wide variety of environmental chemicals, food toxins and drugs (Fig. 3.4.1). Oxidation requires NADPH.

Phase 2. These reactions involve the formation of a covalent link between an exposed functional group on a parent compound with glucuronic acid, sulphate, glutathione, amino acids or acetate. This conjugation process results in a highly polar water-soluble metabolite, which is generally inactive and rapidly excreted into the urine or faeces (Fig. 3.4.1).

The activity of drug-metabolizing enzymes can be altered under various situations that have implications for clinical efficacy.

Induction of CYP. Exposure to certain drugs (e.g. barbiturates) and environmental pollutants (e.g. smoking) induces CYP, resulting in increased drug biotransformation and reduced clinical efficacy. If the metabolite of a particular drug is a reactive species, then induction may be associated with increased toxicity. Many inducers of CYP will also induce enzymes involved in phase 2 reactions (e.g. glutathione transferases).

Competition for drug-metabolizing enzymes. Such competition between two drugs will decrease the metabolism of both drugs and prolong drug activity. One clinically important example of such inhibition is if theophylline is given with a macrolide type antibiotic such as erythromycin, leading to cardiac arrhythmias or seizures.

Inhibition of drug metabolism. Cimetidine, quinidine and ketoconazole all inhibit drug biotransformations. A common mechanism of inhibition of phase 2 reactions involves depletion of the necessary cofactors (e.g. glutathione).

Genetic variation. Small changes in the genetic code (polymorphisms) for enzymes involved in biotransformation can also have an important impact on drug metabolism. Mutations in the gene for CYP2D6 result in a protein that has altered enzyme activity. This has important implications for those individuals who are prescribed

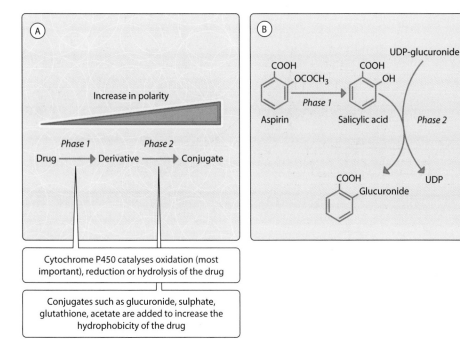

Fig. 3.4.1 Drug metabolism. (A) Phase I and II reactions; (B) example of aspirin metabolism.

cardiovascular agents, psychoactive drugs and morphine derivatives. Similarly, polymorphisms can affect phase 2 reactions; for example 'slow acetylators' would eliminate isoniazid, caffeine and procainamide by N-acetylation more slowly, whereas 'fast acetylators' would require an increased dosage of affected drugs to maintain effective concentrations. The incidence of slow acetylators is 60–70% in Europe.

Drug excretion

Kidney. Both unchanged and biotransformed drugs can be excreted by the kidney. The majority of transformed drug is excreted by the kidney from the renal tubule. The amount of drug entering the tubular lumen is dependent on the amount that is not bound to plasma proteins, the glomerular filtration rate and renal disease. The clearance of creatinine is used as an indicator of impaired renal function. While drug is actively excreted by the kidney, passive reabsorption can occur and this process is influenced by the pH of urine. Alkalization of urine (e.g. with bicarbonate) will result in a greater degree of ionization of a weak acid (e.g. salicylates) within the tubule and reduce its reabsorption.

Increasing urine outflow can also facilitate excretion by reducing the time available for reabsorption.

Gastrointestinal tract. Many drug metabolites formed in the liver are excreted into the intestinal tract in the bile and eliminated in faeces. This is the principal route of excretion for large molecules (e.g. glucuronidation products). Drug conjugate excreted in the bile can undergo hydrolysis by bacteria in the lower intestine, resulting in the release of the parent compound and reabsorption into the circulation (**enterohepatic recirculation**), thus prolonging pharmacological activity. The drug may subsequently be excreted by the kidney (Fig. 3.4.2). In drug overdose, rapid expulsion can be induced by a polyethylene glycol electrolyte lavage, which will induce diarrhoea. Activated charcoal will also slow drug absorption from the gastrointestinal tract.

Lung. Volatile drugs such as general anaesthetics are excreted from the lung. The amount of such substances in exhaled air can be a useful indicator of the level of anaesthesia. While ethanol can be excreted via the lung, this route represents only a fraction of the total elimination of ethanol. Nevertheless, the levels of ethanol in expired air provide a non-invasive measure of blood alcohol levels.

Fig. 3.4.2 Drug movements and enterohepatic recirculation.

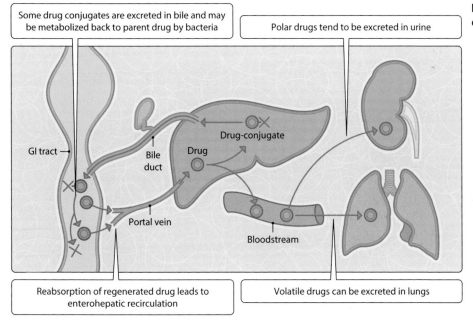

Some drug conjugates are excreted in bile and may be metabolized back to parent drug by bacteria

Polar drugs tend to be excreted in urine

GI tract

Bile duct

Drug

Drug-conjugate

Portal vein

Bloodstream

Reabsorption of regenerated drug leads to enterohepatic recirculation

Volatile drugs can be excreted in lungs

5. Autonomic nervous system

Questions
- What are the major subdivisions of the autonomic nervous system?
- What effect does activation of these systems have on function?

The autonomic nervous system is divided into parasympathetic and sympathetic divisions and these control involuntary activities (see p. 8 and Figs 1.8 and 1.9). Characteristically, autonomic nerves consist of two-neuron chains, with the cell body of the first (preganglionic) lying in the CNS and that of the second (postganglionic) in a ganglion outside the CNS.

Parasympathetic nervous system
The ganglia of the parasympathetic nerves reside within body organs. Preganglionic nerves are generally long while the postganglionic nerves are short, with few interconnections between ganglions and this results in discrete activation of effector cells (see Fig. 1.7).

Activation of the parasympathetic nervous system triggers a cascade of events that ends with a biological response (Fig. 3.5.1).

The release of acetylcholine from preganglionic neurons activates nicotinic receptors on cell bodies of postganglionic neurons within the ganglia. This activation leads to Na^+ entry, membrane depolarization and activation of voltage-dependent sodium channels and it triggers a wave of depolarization along the length of the nerve, ultimately leading to Ca^{2+} entry at the terminal endings via voltage-dependent calcium channels, fusion of acetylcholine vesicles with the plasma membrane and exocytosis of acetylcholine molecules into the neuroeffector junction. Acetylcholine rapidly activates muscarinic receptors on postjunctional membranes of effector cells to evoke a biological response. The release of acetylcholine from these nerve terminals is controlled by prejunctional muscarinic receptors, which limit further release of acetylcholine (negative feedback mechanism). The pharmacological action of acetylcholine is rapidly terminated by the enzyme acetylcholinesterase, which is expressed on the surface of nerve terminals and postsynaptic membranes.

Sympathetic nervous system
The sympathetic system has short preganglionic and long postganglionic nerves. Its ganglia lie close to the spinal column

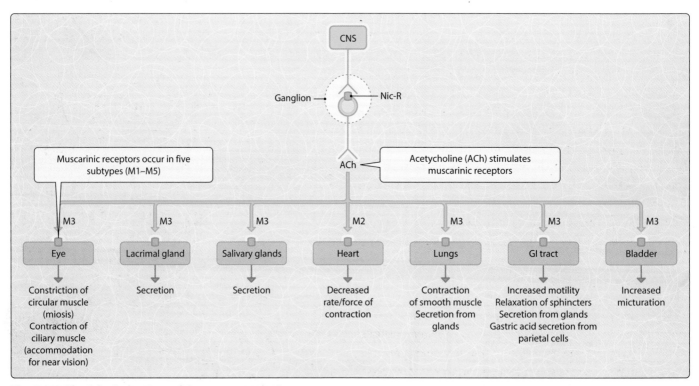

Fig. 3.5.1 Physiological actions of the parasympathetic system.

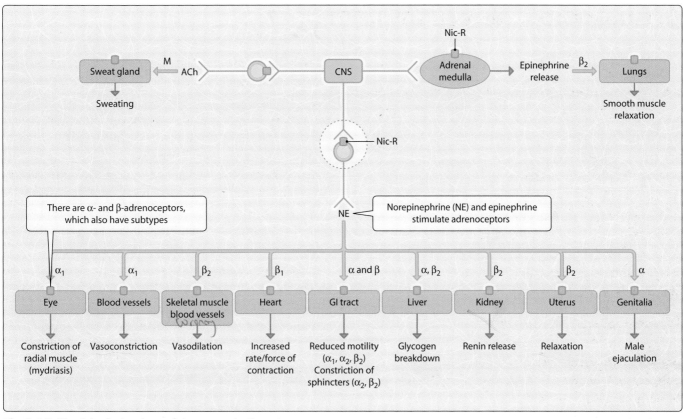

Fig. 3.5.2 Physiological actions of the sympathetic system.

and the two are interconnected. Activation will, therefore, lead to impulses being sent throughout the body, affecting many organs (Fig. 3.5.2).

The activation of the sympathetic nervous system also triggers a series of events; these culminate in the release of norepinephrine from peripheral nerve endings and activation of adrenoceptors on effector cells. The pharmacological action of norepinephrine is terminated by uptake into nerve terminals and either re-packaged in storage vesicles, or metabolism by monoamine oxidase. Adrenoceptors are classified as two major subtypes, α and β, with further subgroupings. The α_1-adrenoceptors are present on cells such as vascular smooth muscle and their activation evokes smooth muscle contraction. The α_2-adrenoceptors exist on prejunctional terminals of the postganglionic sympathetic nerve terminals and their activation results in a negative feedback mechanism to limit further release of norepinephrine. The β-adrenoceptors are present on cardiac tissue and their activation leads to an increase in rate and contractility of the heart.

There are two exceptions with respect to the final neurotransmitter released from sympathetic nerves. Acetylcholine activates nicotinic receptors on chromaffin cells of the adrenal medulla, resulting in the release of epinephrine, a hormone that is released into the general circulation and so will have access to adreno-

ceptors distributed throughout the body. In the skin, acetylcholine released from sympathetic nerves stimulates sweating following activation of muscarinic receptors on sweat glands.

Organs are supplied by both the sympathetic and parasympathetic nervous systems and antagonism between the two systems regulates function (Fig. 3.5.3).

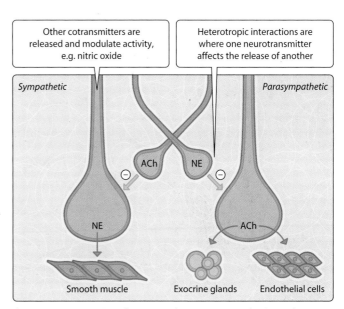

Fig. 3.5.3 Interactions between the parasympathetic and sympathetic systems.

6. Cholinergic neurotransmission

Questions
- What are the pharmacological actions of cholinomimetic agents?
- How does interference with the parasympathetic system affect physiology?

Acetylcholine is synthesized and stored in vesicles and released following activation of voltage-dependent calcium channels (Fig. 3.6.1). The entry of Ca^{2+} into preganglionic nerve terminals triggers the fusion of vesicles with the plasma membrane and release of acetylcholine into the ganglionic junction. This acetylcholine activates the nicotinic receptor (receptor-operated sodium channel) on the postjunctional neuronal membranes within the ganglion. The entry of Na^+ into the postjunctional neuron triggers membrane depolarization, activation of voltage-dependent sodium channels and the propagation of an action potential along the length of the postganglionic nerve,

culminating in the opening of voltage-dependent calcium channels in the terminal endings and the release of acetylcholine into the neuroeffector junction. The release of acetylcholine at neuroeffector sites (e.g. smooth muscle, exocrine glands) activates muscarinic receptors belonging to the G-protein-coupled receptor family. The pharmacological action of acetylcholine is short lived owing to its rapid metabolism by acetylcholinesterase into inactive acetic acid and choline. A variety of drugs can interfere with cholinergic neurotransmission at several sites along this pathway (Fig. 3.6.2).

Cholinomimetic agents

Drugs that mimic the actions of acetylcholine are commonly referred to as cholinomimetic agonists. Muscarinic agonists like **carbachol**, **pilocarpine** and **bethanechol** directly bind to and alter the conformation of muscarinic receptors on effector cells. Acetylcholinesterase inhibitors like **physostigmine** and **neostigmine** are indirect acting stimuli, as they increase the local concentration of acetylcholine at the effector junction by inhibiting acetylcholinesterase.

Cholinomimetics can be used in various clinical situations. Pilocarpine is used to reduce intraocular pressure in patients with glaucoma, while bethanechol is used postoperatively to stimulate the gut and bladder. Neostigmine can be used to reverse skeletal muscle paralysis induced by non-depolarizing neuromuscular blockers. Physostigmine is also used in glaucoma to reduce intraocular pressure. Long-lasting or irreversible acetylcholinesterase inhibitors are used as pesticides (e.g. organophosphates) and in nerve gas (e.g. sarin). Exposure to these agents will induce adverse effects, including bradycardia, hypotension, increased secretions, bronchoconstriction and skeletal muscle paralysis (neuromuscular junction).

Drugs that interfere with parasympathetic neurotransmission

Blocking nicotinic receptors in parasympathetic ganglion with **hexamethonium** can interrupt neurotransmission but this is not a useful action since it does not distinguish between nicotinic receptors of the parasympathetic and sympathetic nervous systems (Ch. 7). Muscarinic antagonists such as **atropine** are non-selective and bind to all muscarinic receptor subtypes, competitively blocking the effect of acetylcholine. Atropine is a tertiary amine and, therefore, lipid soluble; it readily crosses the blood–brain barrier and leads to central excitation (irritability and hyperactivity), hallucination and amnesia. Peripheral actions include, blurred vision, dry mouth,

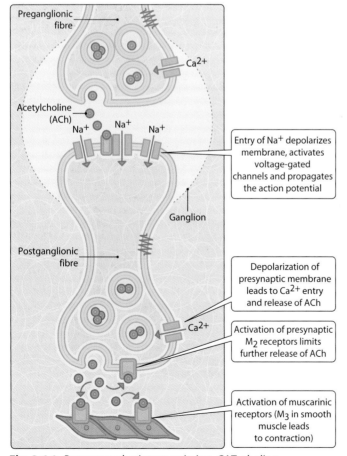

Fig. 3.6.1 Parasympathetic transmission. CAT, choline acetyltransferase; AChE, acetylcholinesterase.

Preganglionic fibre

Acetylcholine (ACh)

Ca^{2+}

Na^+ Na^+ Na^+

Entry of Na^+ depolarizes membrane, activates voltage-gated channels and propagates the action potential

Ganglion

Postganglionic fibre

Ca^{2+}

Depolarization of presynaptic membrane leads to Ca^{2+} entry and release of ACh

Activation of presynaptic M_2 receptors limits further release of ACh

Activation of muscarinic receptors (M_3 in smooth muscle leads to contraction)

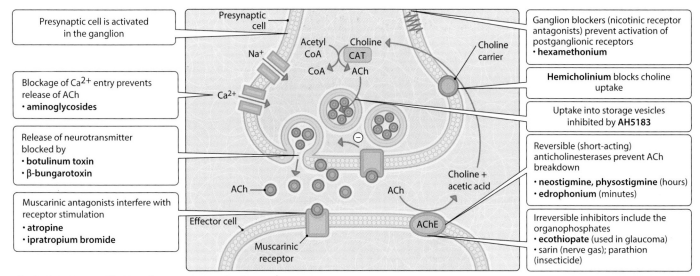

Fig. 3.6.2 Drugs affecting the parasympathetic system.

reduced secretions, increased body temperature (inhibition of sweat glands), paralysis of accommodation and urinary retention. Atropine can be used to treat poisoning with organophosphates to minimize the peripheral autonomic action of excessive acetylcholine stimulation but it will have no effect in reversing skeletal muscle paralysis. Because the quaternary amines are charged at physiological pH, they have a better safety profile. They are used in the treatment of respiratory diseases such as asthma and chronic obstructive pulmonary disease (e.g.

ipratropium bromide), where they cause bronchodilatation by blocking vagal activation of the airway smooth muscle. Drugs like **hyoscine** (non-selective) are used to treat motion sickness, **tropicamide** (M_4 selective) to cause pupil dilatation, **pirenzepine** (M_1 selective) to reduce gastric acid secretion, **benzhexol** (M_1 selective) in Parkinson's disease, and to terodine (M_3 selective) in urinary incontinence. Muscarinic antagonists can be used in anaesthesia to prevent bronchial secretions and vagal slowing of heart rate.

7. Sympathetic neurotransmission

Questions
- What are the pharmacological actions of sympathomimetics?
- How does interference with the sympathetic system affect physiology?

The action potential in the postganglionic fibre is generated in the same manner as described in Ch. 6 for the parasympathetic ganglion (Fig. 3.7.1). Here, however, the postganglionic nerve terminal contains enzymes necessary for the synthesis of norepinephrine from L-tyrosine. Norepinephrine is stored in vesicles and released following activation of voltage-dependent calcium channels. The entry of Ca^{2+} into the nerve terminal triggers the fusion of vesicles with plasma membrane and release of norepinephrine molecules into the neuroeffector junction. The pharmacological action of norepinephrine is short lived, owing to its rapid uptake into sympathetic nerve terminals and either

repackaging into storage vesicle or metabolism by the enzyme **monoamine oxidase** (MAO) to 3-methoxy-4-hydroxymandelic acid. The release of norepinephrine at neuroeffector sites (e.g. vascular smooth muscle) results in activation of adrenoceptors that belong to the family of G-protein-coupled receptors. A variety of drugs can interfere with sympathetic neurotransmission at several sites along this pathway (Fig. 3.7.2). Epinephrine is released from the adrenal glands into the circulation and also acts on α- and β-adrenoceptors on effector cells. It is rapidly metabolized by **catechol-*O*-methyltransferase** (COMT) and MAO in the liver and gut wall.

Adrenoceptor agonists
Drugs that mimic the actions of norepinephrine and epinephrine are commonly referred to as sympathomimetics. Epinephrine (adrenaline) is used in emergency situations for acute treatment of anaphylactic shock. The effect of norepinephrine and epinephrine on the cardiovascular system is complex. Norepinephrine stimulates vascular smooth muscle contraction ($α_1$-adrenoceptor), resulting in an increase in total peripheral resistance, which will activate reflex slowing of the heart, thereby negating the direct action of norepinephrine on cardiac $β_1$-adrenoceptors. Epinephrine can increase rate and force of contraction (β-adrenoceptor) but also stimulate vasoconstriction ($α_1$-adrenoceptor). Total peripheral resistance may actually fall because of the vasodilator effect of epinephrine on arterioles supplying skeletal muscle ($β_2$-adrenoceptors).

Alpha-adrenoceptor agonists like **clonidine** ($α_2$-adrenoceptor) selectively inhibit further release of norepinephrine from nerve terminals and are used in the treatment of hypertension. **Phenylephrine** ($α_1$-adrenoceptor) contracts vascular smooth muscle and is used in acute hypotension and as a nasal decongestant. Drugs like **isoprenaline** (non-selective), **salbutamol** ($β_2$-adrenoceptor) and **dobutamine** ($β_1$-adrenoceptor) are direct stimulants of β-adrenoceptors. They are used to treat heart block (isoprenaline) and congestive heart failure (dobutamine). Beta-adrenoceptor drugs like **salbutamol**, **terbutaline**, **salmeterol** and **formoterol** ($β_2$-adrenoceptor) are powerful relaxants of airway smooth muscle and cause bronchodilatation; they are used for the symptomatic treatment of asthma and chronic obstructive pulmonary disease.

Indirect acting stimuli such as tyramine (contained in cheese, wines), **ephedrine** (nasal decongestant) and **amphetamine** (substance of abuse) release norepinephrine from storage vesicles and stimulate $α_1$-adrenoceptors on vascular smooth

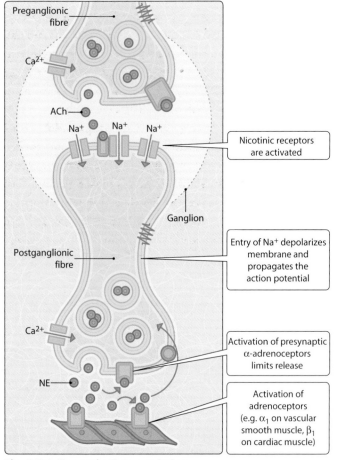

Fig. 3.7.1 Sympathetic transmission.

Labels in figure:
- Preganglionic fibre
- Ca^{2+}
- ACh
- Na^+ Na^+ Na^+
- Nicotinic receptors are activated
- Ganglion
- Entry of Na^+ depolarizes membrane and propagates the action potential
- Postganglionic fibre
- Ca^{2+}
- Activation of presynaptic α-adrenoceptors limits release
- NE
- Activation of adrenoceptors (e.g. $α_1$ on vascular smooth muscle, $β_1$ on cardiac muscle)

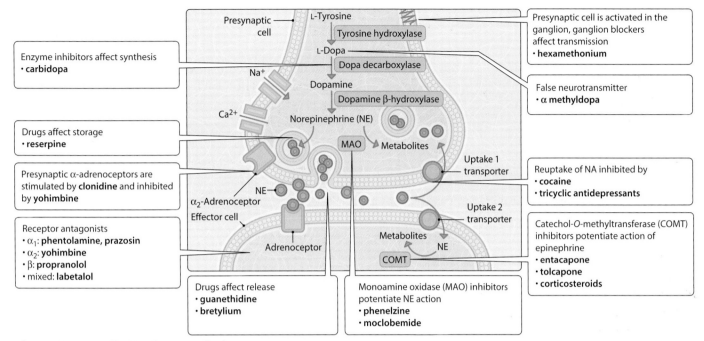

Fig. 3.7.2 Drugs affecting the sympathetic system.

Image labels:

Presynaptic cell

L-Tyrosine
Tyrosine hydroxylase
L-Dopa
Dopa decarboxylase
Dopamine
Dopamine β-hydroxylase
Norepinephrine (NE)
MAO → Metabolites

Na⁺
Ca²⁺

NE
α₂-Adrenoceptor
Effector cell
Adrenoceptor

Uptake 1 transporter
Uptake 2 transporter
Metabolites
NE
COMT

Enzyme inhibitors affect synthesis
• carbidopa

Drugs affect storage
• reserpine

Presynaptic α-adrenoceptors are stimulated by clonidine and inhibited by yohimbine

Receptor antagonists
• α₁: phentolamine, prazosin
• α₂: yohimbine
• β: propranolol
• mixed: labetalol

Presynaptic cell is activated in the ganglion, ganglion blockers affect transmission
• hexamethonium

False neurotransmitter
• α methyldopa

Reuptake of NA inhibited by
• cocaine
• tricyclic antidepressants

Catechol-O-methyltransferase (COMT) inhibitors potentiate action of epinephrine
• entacapone
• tolcapone
• corticosteroids

Drugs affect release
• guanethidine
• bretylium

Monoamine oxidase (MAO) inhibitors potentiate NE action
• phenelzine
• moclobemide

---

muscle cells, leading to hypertension and severe headache, which can be exacerbated in subjects who take MAO inhibitors.

Drugs that interfere with sympathetic neurotransmission

There are a number of potential sites along the sympathetic nerve where drugs act to alter neurotransmission (Fig. 3.7.2) and their pharmacology will be described in greater detail in Ch. 8. Blocking nicotinic receptors in sympathetic ganglion with **hexamethonium** can interrupt neurotransmission but does so in both parasympathetic and sympathetic systems. Non-selective α-adrenoceptor antagonists like **phentolamine** block α₁-adrenoceptors on vascular smooth muscle, causing a fall in blood pressure and postural hypotension. This leads to reflex tachycardia, which is exacerbated since cardiac prejunctional

α₂-adrenoceptors are also blocked, resulting in increased release of norepinephrine in the heart and overstimulation of cardiac β-adrenoceptors (not blocked). Other side-effects include nasal congestion, impotence and diarrhoea. The α₁-selective antagonist **prazosin** is used in the treatment of hypertension but also causes postural hypotension, albeit without the exaggerated reflex tachycardia (α₂-adrenoceptors not blocked). These drugs can also be used in the diagnosis of phaeochromocytoma, a tumour of the secretory cells of the adrenal medulla.

Beta-adrenoceptor antagonists like **propranolol** (non-selective), **practolol** and **metoprolol** (β₁-selective) are used in the treatment of hypertension, cardiac arrhythmias and angina pectoris. **Timolol** (β₁-selective) is used to reduce glaucoma but is contraindicated in subjects with asthma as it will precipitate an exacerbation of symptoms. **Labetalol** is a non-selective α- and β-adrenoceptor antagonist and is used in hypertension.

8. Neuromuscular junction

Questions
- How is skeletal muscle function regulated?
- What pharmacological agents can interfere with this process?

Physiology of the neuromuscular junction

Skeletal (voluntary) muscle receives a rich supply of fast-conducting motor neurons containing acetylcholine in their terminals. Depolarization releases acetylcholine, which diffuses across the neuromuscular junction (NMJ); two molecules bind to the two α-subunits of the nicotinic receptor on the motor end-plate region, leading to depolarization of the motor end plate and contraction of skeletal muscle cells. Acetylcholine is also rapidly metabolized by acetycholinesterase into inactive choline and acetic acid; the choline is reincorporated into the terminals of the motor neurons and converted back to acetylcholine by the enzyme choline acetyltransferase (Fig. 3.8.1). The opening (approximately 1 ms) of the nicotinic receptor allows the entry of Na^+ into the cell, resulting in a brief depolarization; this is known as the end plate potential. If this is of sufficient stimulus to reach threshold, the resultant action potential leads to the depolarization of adjacent skeletal muscle cells via depolarization of many other voltage-dependent sodium channels. This wave spreads over the muscle surface and is conducted within the interior of the fibre by invaginations (T-tubules) in the muscle cell. The action potential leads to the release of Ca^{2+} from the sarcoplasmic reticulum, which is in close proximity to the T-tubules, and ultimately triggers skeletal muscle contraction (Fig. 3.8.2).

Pharmacological modulation

Uptake of choline. The rate-limiting step in the synthesis of acetylcholine is the transport of choline back into nerve terminals. **Hemicholinium**, which is an analogue of choline, blocks this transporter, leading to slow depletion of acetylcholine from storage vesicles. It is of little clinical utility since the depletion is dependent upon the frequency of nerve stimulation. AH5183 is a drug that inhibits the active transport of acetylcholine into storage vesicles.

Exocytosis of acetylcholine. Since Ca^{2+} entry is required to promote the release of acetylcholine from storage vesicles, agents that interfere with Ca^{2+} entry will inhibit acetylcholine release. Aminoglycoside antibiotics (e.g. **streptomycin**) block this exocytosis and can lead to muscle paralysis, which can be reversed by supplementation with calcium salts. The anaerobic bacillus *Clostridium botulinum* produces a neurotoxin, botulinum toxin, that interferes with the exocytosis mechanism, as does β-bungarotoxin in snake venom. Food poisoning by *C. botulinum* will lead to muscle paralysis and interfere with parasympathetic transmission (Ch. 6). Botulinum toxin type A is used in cosmetic surgery to induce muscle paralysis in the face or in conditions where there is excessive muscle contraction (e.g. dystonias).

Competitive inhibitors. Inhibition of acetylcholine binding to the nicotinic receptor can also interfere with neurotransmission. Non-depolarizing neuromuscular blockers (e.g. **tubocurarine**, **gallamine**, **pancuronium**, **vecuronium** and **atracurium**) bind in a competitive manner to the skeletal muscle nicotinic receptor to induce muscle paralysis, which offers obvious advantages in surgery (Fig. 3.8.2B). These quaternary amines do not cross the blood–brain barrier and have poor oral bioavailability (so are given i.v.). The blockade can be reversed by increasing the local concentration of acetylcholine in the NMJ using an acetylcholinesterase inhibitor. Some of these agents have several side-effects, including histamine release from mast cells and ganglion blockage (tubocurarine, atracurium) or muscarinic receptor antagonism that can lead to tachycardia (pancuronium, gallamine). **Rocuronium** is a

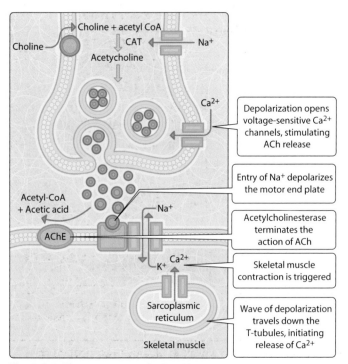

Fig. 3.8.1 The neuromuscular junction.

Choline + acetyl CoA

Choline —

CAT ← Na^+

Acetycholine

Ca^{2+}

Depolarization opens voltage-sensitive Ca^{2+} channels, stimulating ACh release

Acetyl-CoA + Acetic acid

AChE

Na^+

Entry of Na^+ depolarizes the motor end plate

Acetylcholinesterase terminates the action of ACh

K^+ Ca^{2+}

Skeletal muscle contraction is triggered

Sarcoplasmic reticulum

Skeletal muscle

Wave of depolarization travels down the T-tubules, initiating release of Ca^{2+}

short-acting blocker that has no reported cardiovascular side-effects.

Depolarizing blockers. **Suxamethonium** (succinylcholine) is a depolarizing neuromuscular blocker with rapid onset and short duration of action. It initially binds to the receptor for a longer period than acetylcholine since it is not metabolized by acetylcholinesterase in the NMJ (it is metabolized by plasma cholinesterases). The resulting activation of the nicotinic receptor and surrounding voltage-dependent sodium channels initially activates skeletal muscle contraction (fasciculation). Persistent stimulation with suxamethonium leads to muscle paralysis through occupation of the nicotinic receptors, thus preventing binding of acetylcholine and subsequent activation of the receptor and surrounding voltage-dependent sodium channels (Fig. 3.8.2C).

Acetylcholinesterase inhibitors. Blockage of the enzyme responsible for terminating the action of acetylcholine will increase the duration of its action in the NMJ (Fig. 3.8.2D). Drugs like **edrophonium, neostigmine** and **pyridostigmine**

are quaternary amines that inhibit acetylcholinesterase but differ in their duration of action. This depends on the nature of binding of these inhibitors to the enzyme. Edrophonium is short acting (minutes) and is quickly hydrolysed by the enzyme (but slower than hydrolysis of acetylcholine). Neostigmine forms a more stable bond with the enzyme and is more slowly hydrolysed (hours); it can be given to reverse the effects of a non-depolarizing NMJ blocker. A muscarinic antagonist may be employed to counteract the resultant overactivity of the parasympathetic nervous system owing to inhibition of acetylcholinesterase in these nerves. These inhibitors (neostigmine, pyridostigmine) are also used in myasthenia gravis, an autoimmune disease characterized by muscle weakness as a result of loss of functional nicotinic receptors in the muscle end plate. Since autoantibodies (IgG) are responsible for this loss, treatment with glucocorticosteroids (e.g. prednisolone), immunosuppressants (e.g. azathioprine) and thymectomy may also be employed to downregulate the immune system and prevent the formation of these autoantibodies.

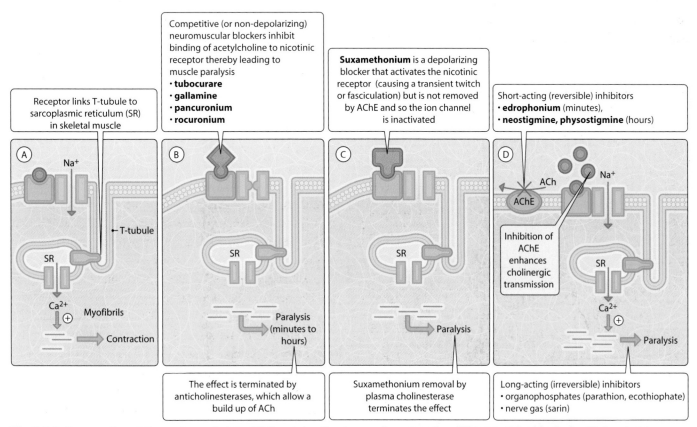

Fig. 3.8.2 Drugs acting at the motor end plate. (A) Events leading to muscle contraction; (B) competitive blockade; (C) depolarizing blockade; (D) anticholinesterases.

9. Local anaesthetics

Questions
- How are nerve impulses produced?
- What is the mechanism of action of local anaesthetics?

Nerve conduction

The lipid membrane provides a physical barrier for the movement of ions between the extracellular and intracellular domains of cells including neuronal cells. The Na^+/K^+-ATPase pump is an energy-dependent protein that pumps Na^+ out of cells and K^+ into cells thereby creating an electrochemical gradient and a resting membrane potential of −70 mV. Opening of voltage-dependent sodium channels leads to an influx of Na^+ into the cell (e.g. nerve) and a rise of membrane potential; this leads to the opening of neighbouring voltage-dependent sodium channels. Once a threshold of 15 mV or greater has been reached, an action potential is generated that results in a wave of depolarization along the length of the nerve. The sodium channel then closes and is refractory to further opening (inactivated state). The membrane hyperpolarizes when potassium channels open, allowing K^+ to flow out of the cell and the nerve is refractory to further stimulation. The Na^+/K^+-ATPase pump then restores membrane potential back to −70 mV and the sodium channel reverts from a refractory to a closed state that is able to be opened by new changes in membrane potential (Fig. 3.9.1). The

sodium channel has four domains (D_1–D_4) each containing six membrane-spanning helices (S1–S6). The S4 membrane-spanning helix of each domain contains positively charged amino acids and serves as a voltage sensor. The S5 and S6 spanning helices are connected by a short membrane-associated loop that serves as the outer pore of the channel, selectively gating for Na^+. A short intracellular loop connects S3 and S4 and contains the amino acid sequence isoleucine–phenylephrine–methionine (IMF), which functions as an inactivation gate. The IMF particle is thought to insert into the intracellular mouth of the channel pore and, by binding to a specific site, prevents the entry of Na^+ (Fig. 3.9.1).

Pharmacology of local anaesthetics

Local anaesthetics are weak bases (pK_A 8–9) and only the uncharged form of the drug can penetrate the lipid membrane (Fig. 3.9.2). Local anaesthetics block sodium channels and nerve conduction by binding to specific amino acid sequences located within the pore domain of the ion channel (Fig. 3.9.3A). These sequences are found near the centre and proximal to the intracellular domain of the cell (Fig. 3.9.3B). The uncharged form of the local anaesthetic diffuses across the lipid membrane and becomes charged once inside the intracellular domain of the cell. The drug requires that the channel is open for cumulative binding. Therefore, inhibition of the sodium channel by a local anaesthetic is often described as use dependent. A number of toxins are

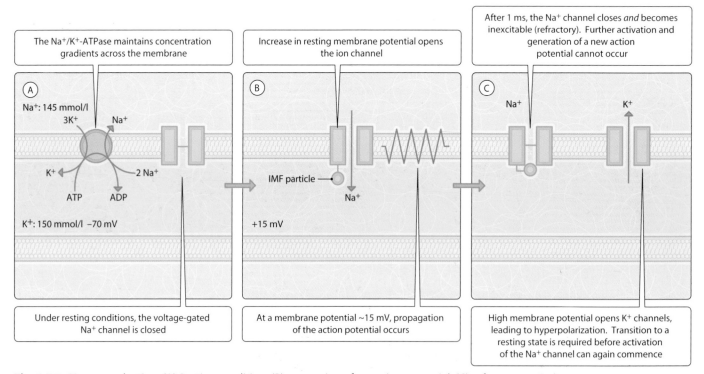

Fig. 3.9.1 Nerve conduction. (A) Resting condition; (B) generation of an action potential; (C) refractory period.

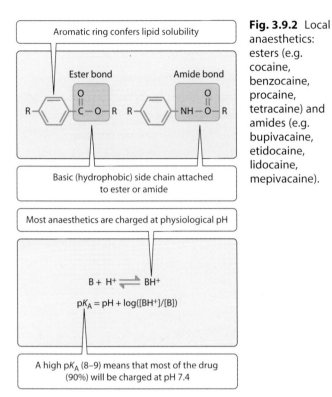

Fig. 3.9.2 Local anaesthetics: esters (e.g. cocaine, benzocaine, procaine, tetracaine) and amides (e.g. bupivacaine, etidocaine, lidocaine, mepivacaine).

Local anaesthetics are composed of an aromatic group (lipophilic end) linked to a basic side chain by an ester or amide group (Fig. 3.9.2). Ester-based drugs are inactivated by plasma cholinesterases while amides are metabolized in the liver. The duration of action of a local anaesthetic is also dependent upon the drug's lipophilicity: the greater the lipid solubility the longer is the retention time of the molecule within the neuronal membrane. **Bupivacaine** is more lipid soluble than **lidocaine** and has a greater duration of action. Another factor that will reduce clinical efficacy is the rate of removal of the drug from the site of injection. Coinjecting the local anaesthetic with epinephrine, which promotes vasoconstriction, prolongs duration of action.

Local anaesthetics are effective in blocking conduction in small nerve fibre types, particularly those involved in pain perception, while larger fibres are affected to a lesser extent. Small fibres have a greater ratio of surface area to volume than larger fibres and so will preferentially accumulate local anaesthetic. Local anaesthetics are routinely used in ophthalmology (**tetracaine**, **proparacaine**), applied to mucosal surfaces (benzocaine, lidocaine) and used for spinal and epidural anaesthesia (bupivacaine).

known to block sodium channels (e.g. tetrodotoxin) by binding to its extracellular pore domain. In contrast, quaternary local anaesthetics like QX314 can only block the channel when applied to the intracellular surface of the channel. An exception to this rule is **benzocaine**, which is an uncharged local anaesthetic that weakly binds to the sodium channel. It presumably gains access via the lipid bilayer as the inhibition is not use dependent.

A number of unwanted side-effects are characteristic of this drug class and include irritation and inflammation at the site of injection. Hypoxia can result when local anaesthetics are coinjected with α_1-adrenoceptor agonists. High systemic doses may affect excitable tissues of the heart, causing cardiotoxicity, and within the CNS, giving rise to restlessness, tremor and convulsion. Central stimulation is followed by depression.

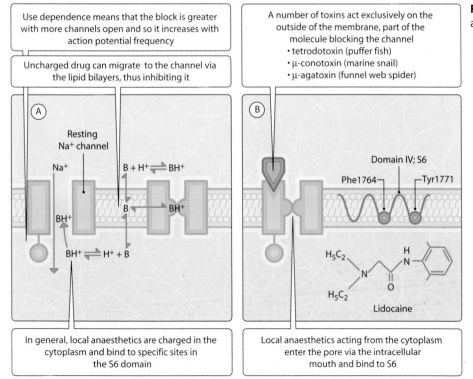

Fig. 3.9.3 The effect of local anaesthetics and toxins on sodium channels.

10. Arrhythmias

Questions
- How are action potentials generated in the heart?
- What causes arrhythmias?
- How do anti-arrhythmia drugs act?

Cardiac electrophysiology

The rhythmicity of the heart is controlled by the sinoatrial (SA) node, which constantly fires (70–80 discharges/min; faster than any other region in the heart). Action potentials generated in this node quickly travel throughout the atria and ventricles via the atrioventricular (AV) node, which connects the two areas electrically; action potentials spread down the right and left side of the bundle of His, which connects with Purkinje fibres conducting impulses throughout the ventricular muscle mass. Both parasympathetic (decrease) and sympathetic (increase) nervous systems influence action potential discharge from the SA node. Action potentials generated in the SA node and ventricular cells are characterized by the opening of different ion channels, and the shape and time course of the action potentials generated are dependent upon the types of ion channel involved (Fig. 3.10.1).

Arrhythmias can result from abnormal impulse generation or conduction. Myocardial infarction (MI) is a major predisposing factor for ventricular arrhythmias. Impaired blood flow to ventricular muscle in atherosclerosis can give rise to hypoxia and MI. Arrhythmias are classified according to their origin:

- delayed after-depolarization, inward current associated with raised intracellular Ca^{2+} triggers ectopic beats
- re-entry, resulting from partial conduction block (parts of the myocardium are depolarized); conduction then depends on slow Ca^{2+} current
- ectopic pacemaker activity, encouraged by sympathetic activity
- heart block resulting from damage to the AV node or ventricular conducting system.

Clinically, arrhythmias are divided according to their site of origin (supraventricular (SA node, atria, AV node) and ventricular) and according to whether the heart rate is increased or decreased (tachycardia or bradycardia).

Treatment of arrhythmias

The implantation of electrical pacemakers, electrical defibrillation and surgery are non-pharmacological alternatives for the

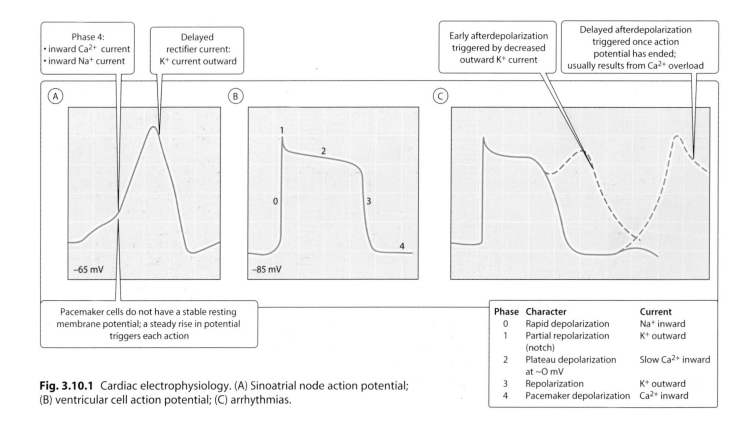

Fig. 3.10.1 Cardiac electrophysiology. (A) Sinoatrial node action potential; (B) ventricular cell action potential; (C) arrhythmias.

Phase	Character	Current
0	Rapid depolarization	Na^+ inward
1	Partial repolarization (notch)	K^+ outward
2	Plateau depolarization at ~0 mV	Slow Ca^{2+} inward
3	Repolarization	K^+ outward
4	Pacemaker depolarization	Ca^{2+} inward

treatment of arrhythmias. Anti-arrhythmic drugs are classified by the Vaughn Williams classification (Table 3.10.1) based upon their effects on the action potential.

Class I drugs block the inward depolarizing Na^+ current (phase 0), slowing depolarization rate and reducing cell excitability. They bind to sodium channels in the open or refractory state. Consequently, the more frequently the channels are activated, the greater the degree of block ('use dependence') and action is preferentially during high-frequency stimulation of the heart in arrhythmia, not in the normal beating heart. Subgroups are based on the speed of association and dissociation from the channels. **Class Ia** drugs are the oldest group and they block sodium channels in the open (activated) state, slow the rate of rise in the depolarizing phase of the action potential and prolong the refractory period. **Class Ib** drugs associate and dissociate rapidly during the normal heartbeat but prevent the development of a premature beat because they will block the channels at this point (i.e. preference for refractory channels). **Class Ic** drugs associate and dissociate very slowly, thus reaching a steady-state level of block, and depress conduction. However, they are contraindicated in patients with MI as they have a pro-arrhythmic effect.

Class II decrease the rate of depolarization of SA and AV nodes by inhibiting sympathetic drive to the heart and are of particular use when exercise and stress are precipitating factors in susceptible individuals.

Class III drugs prolong the duration of the action potential but have no effect on conduction velocity and delay repolarization. **Bretylium** blocks potassium channels; it also has adrenergic blocking effects, which explains its adverse effects. **Amiodarone** is a non-selective agent blocking potassium, sodium and calcium channels and inhibiting α- and β-adrenoceptors. **Sotalol** is a mixed class II/III inhibitor and inhibition of β-adrenoceptors and potassium channels may account for its clinical efficacy.

Class IV drugs block calcium channels (L-type; phase 2) and so decrease the conduction velocity of SA and AV nodes where depolarization is dependent upon opening of these channels.

Other drugs include **atropine** (sinus bradycardia), **epinephrine** (adrenaline) (cardiac arrest), **isoprenaline** (heart block), **calcium chloride** (ventricular tachycardia owing to hyperkalaemia) and **magnesium chloride** (ventricular fibrillation, digoxin toxicity). **Adenosine** activates adenosine A_1 receptors in SA and AV nodes, which leads to a hyperpolarizing K^+ current (supraventricular tachycardia). **Digoxin** blocks Na^+/K^+-ATPase, facilitating acetylcholine release from the vagus nerve, shortening atrial refractory period and slowing conduction in the AV node (rapid atrial fibrillation).

Table 3.10.1 ANTI-ARRHYTHMIA DRUGS

Class	Example(s)	Clinical uses	Adverse effects
Ia	Disopyramide	V arrhythmias; prevention of recurrent paroxysmal atrial fibrillation triggered by vagal overactivity	Anticholinergic effects
Ib	Lidocaine	V tachycardia and fibrillation during and immediately after myocardial infarction	CNS effects (drowsiness, disorientation and convulsions), hypotension, bradycardia
1c	Flecainide	As 1a, plus WP	Nausea, vomiting, CNS toxicity, negative inotrophy
II	Beta-adrenoceptor antagonists (propranolol, atenolol)	SV and V arrhythmias; reduce mortality following myocardial infarction; prevent recurrence of tachyarrhythmias provoked by increased sympathetic activity	Bronchospasm, fatigue, insomnia, dizziness, bradycardia, hypotension, decreased glucose tolerance in diabetics
III	Amiodarone, bretylium, sotalol, ibutilide	SV and V tachycardia, including WPW (amiodarone); paroxysmal SV arrhythmias, suppression ventricular ectopic beats and ventricular tachycardia (sotalol)	Amiodarone: photosensitivity, thyroid dysfunction, pulmonary fibrosis (slow onset but may be irreversible), corneal deposits, liver dysfunction. Sotalol, bretylium: hypotension, nausea, vomiting
IV	Verapamil	Prevents recurrence of paroxysmal SV tachycardia; reduces ventricular rate in atrial fibrillation	Hypotension, rash, bradycardia, heart block, constipation

V, ventricular; SV, supraventricular; WPW, Wolff–Parkinson–White syndrome

11. Angina pectoris

Questions
- What is angina pectoris?
- How is it treated?

Pathophysiology

The coronary arteries provide myocardial smooth muscle with a rich blood supply to meet its oxygen demand. However, if demand cannot be satisfied, myocardial ischaemia ensues, which presents as a radiating chest pain. **Stable angina** (classic angina) is a consequence of a fixed obstruction of the coronary arteries and is triggered by stress or exercise. **Unstable angina** (precipitated by coronary thrombosis) can occur suddenly at rest with increasing severity and frequency of attacks. **Variant angina** is usually the result of coronary artery spasm and is accompanied by chest pain and ventricular arrhythmias. Diseases causing angina include coronary atherosclerosis, transient platelet aggregation and coronary thrombosis, coronary vasospasm owing to sympathetic stimulation and endothelial cell damage, and accumulation of vasoconstrictors. A variety of pharmacological agents are used in the treatment of angina:

- reducing preload by dilating veins (capacitance vessels): organic nitrates (vasodilatation)
- reducing heart rate and contractility: beta-blockers, calcium channel blockers
- increasing blood supply to the heart by coronary artery vasodilatation: dipyramidole
- reducing afterload by dilating arteries (resistance vessels): calcium channel blockers, organic nitrates
- preventing coronary thrombosis: aspirin.

Treatment of angina

Organic nitrates

Glyceryltrinitrate (GTN), **nitroglycerin**, **isosorbide mononitrate** (ISM) and **isosorbide dinitrate** (IDN) are prodrugs (nitrovasodilators) that are biotransformed within vascular smooth muscle cells via various enzymatic reactions (e.g. mitochondrial aldehyde dehydrogenase, cytochrome P450) to yield nitric oxide, which activates soluable guanylyl cyclase thereby stimulating vasodilatation (Fig. 3.11.1). The major action of organic nitrates is venodilatation (capacitance vessels), thereby reducing venous return and preload to the heart. This will reduce myocardial wall tension, oxygen demand, ischaemia and hence pain. Organic nitrates have little vasodilating activity on coronary arteries, particularly if atherosclerosis is present and obstruction is fixed. Vasodilatation of collateral vessels may increase blood flow to the myocardium. While not a major action, nitrates can also reduce total peripheral resistance following dilatation of arterioles (resistance vessels). However, sympathetic reflexes overcome any benefit derived from this mechanism.

Nitroglycerin is administered by the sublingual route in order to avoid first pass metabolism and acts within minutes for the treatment of acute angina. The other nitrates are used in stable angina to prevent attacks and may be administered orally or by patches applied to the skin. Adverse effects of nitrovasodilators include postural hypotension, dizziness, tachycardia, flushing and headache. With prolonged use, tolerance can develop, which may be minimized by alternating between different formulations. This drug class can be used in combination with β-adrenoceptor antagonists or calcium channel blockers.

Beta-blockers

Norepinephrine released from sympathetic terminals innervating the heart (or epinephrine released from adrenal medulla) increases force and rate of contraction by stimulating cardiac β-adrenoceptors. This increases oxygen demand. Beta-blockers bind to cardiac β_1-adrenoceptors and prevent norepinephrine binding. This reduces sympathetic input to the SA node, thereby reducing the excitability of pacemaker cells (Fig. 3.11.2).

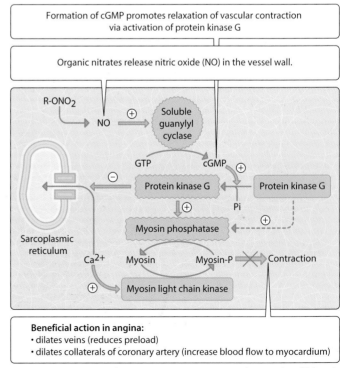

Fig. 3.11.1 Action of organic nitrates in smooth muscle of blood vessels.

Beta-blockers are used prophylactically to treat angina. Drugs such as **propranolol** and the more β_1-selective drugs like **atenolol** are administered orally and are taken prophylactically for the treatment of stable angina. Side-effects include bronchospasm (so are contraindicated in asthma), fatigue, insomnia, dizziness, bradycardia, heart block (contraindicated in patients with AV block), hypotension and decreased glucose tolerance in diabetes.

Calcium channel antagonists

The calcium channel antagonists (e.g. **verapamil** (phenethylalkylamine), **diltiazem** (dibenzazepine) and the 1,4-dihydropyridines (e.g. **nifedipine**) inhibit Ca^{2+} entry by blocking the opening of L-type calcium channels in cardiac and vascular smooth muscle (Fig. 3.11.3). Changes in vascular smooth muscle reduces afterload, and increased coronary blood flow improves oxygen availability. Reduced cardiac contractility and heart rate also reduce myocardial oxygen consumption. Verapamil and diltiazem inhibit calcium channels in heart muscle and so have a negative inotropic action. In contrast, nifedipine is not effective against cardiac calcium channels, appearing to be selective for vascular smooth muscle cells. Consequently, it causes vasodilatation without altering AV conduction, myocardial contractility or heart rate.

Calcium channel blockers are administered orally for the treatment of stable angina. The systemic vasodilatation induced by nifedipine may cause dizziness, palpitation, flushing, reflex tachycardia and oedema. The major side-effects of verapamil include bradycardia, hypotension, heart block and constipation and it is, therefore, contraindicated in patients with heart failure, AV block, bradycardia or hypotension.

Other treatments

Dipyridamol. Used for the treatment of unstable angina, it prevents the uptake/metabolism of adenosine, an endogenous vasodilator. Adenosine accumulation within arteriolar smooth muscle leads to dilatation and is particularly useful in unstable variant angina caused by coronary artery spasm. This drug is also a non-selective phosphodiesterase inhibitor, thereby promoting cyclic nucleotide levels in cells and relaxation of smooth muscle. Side-effects include nausea, diarrhoea, hypotension and headache.

Aspirin. Aspirin is a non-selective cyclooxygenase (COX) inhibitor and so reduces the synthesis of platelet-derived thromboxane A_2, a powerful vasoconstrictor and aggregator of platelets. Aspirin will also inhibit the production of endothelial cell-derived prostaglandin I_2 (prostacyclin), which is a vasodilator and inhibitor of platelet aggregation. This inhibition of COX within the endothelium is short lived because of de novo synthesis of this protein. However, platelet COX is inhibited for the duration of the circulating life-time of this cell (7–10 days) because platelets are enucleated and do not have the capacity to synthesize proteins. Platelet aggregation and coronary thrombosis can precipitate unstable angina, so aspirin can reduce the incidence of coronary thrombosis rather than specifically treating angina. Side-effects include gastric bleeding, ulceration with overdose, reduced renal function owing to reduced renal blood flow and bronchospasm in asthma.

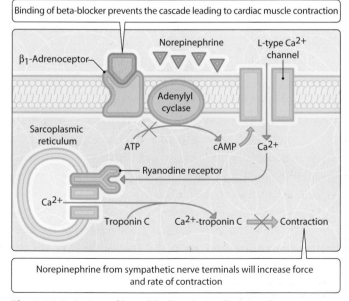

Fig. 3.11.2 Action of beta-blockers in cardiac muscle.

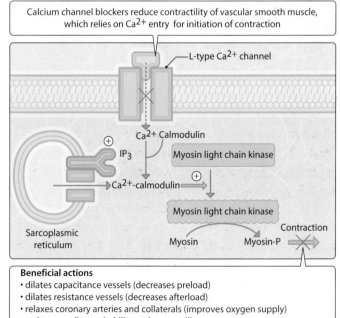

Fig. 3.11.3 Action of calcium channel blockers in vascular smooth muscle.

12. Congestive heart failure

Questions
- What is congestive heart failure?
- What drugs are used in congestive heart failure?

Pathophysiology

Congestive heart failure (CHF) is a failure of the ventricles to maintain adequate output and has many causes, including myocardial infarction, hypertension and cardiomyopathies. In backward failure, blood is not efficiently pumped out of the ventricles. This leads to an increase in ventricular filling pressure, giving rise to venous congestion and systemic oedema (Fig. 3.12.1). In forward failure, the fall in cardiac ouput means that less blood reaches the kidneys and this stimulates Na^+ and water retention, which exacerbates further fluid retention and systemic oedema (see Fig. 1.13). Fluid retention in the lung owing to increased pressure in the veins in the lung results in shortness of breath and pulmonary oedema. Weakness and fatigue are symptoms associated with lower blood supply to other organs. The body attempts to compensate by stimulating extrahumoral (sympathetic) reflexes to restore cardiac output by increasing cardiac contractility and vasoconstriction (Fig. 3.12.2). The heart is forced to pump against an increasing resistance (afterload), which depresses cardiac output. The fall in blood supply to the kidney again increases venous return (preload) and tissue oedema. This increase in preload contributes to the incomplete emptying of the ventricles and a rise in end-diastolic pressure. This activates an intrinsic cardiac compensatory mechanism and as ventricular hypertrophy develops this may reduce tension generated by the muscle (Frank–Starling curve) and the heart eventually fails.

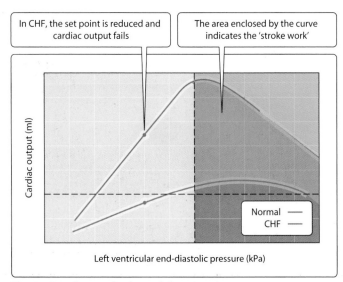

Fig. 3.12.1 Congestive heart failure (CHF).

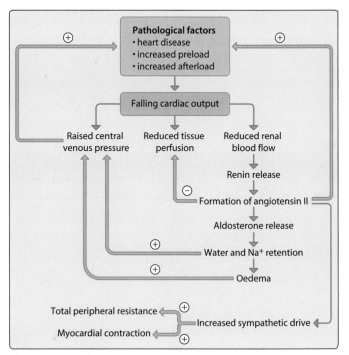

Fig. 3.12.2 Pathogenesis of heart failure.

Drug treatment

Drug therapy may improve cardiac contractility (positive inotropes, cardiac glycosides, phosphodiesterase 3 (PDE3) inhibitors, β_1-adrenoceptor agonists) or reduce preload and congestion (diuretics, angiotensin-converting enzyme (ACE) inhibitors, nitrovasodilators), having different effects on smooth and cardiac muscle (Figs 3.12.3 and 3.12.4).

Cardiac contractility

Cardiac glycosides. **Digoxin** is the prototypical cardiac glycoside (Fig. 3.12.3). Cardiac glycosides inhibit the Na^+/K^+-ATPase energy pump so Na^+ accumulates within myocardial cells. This reduces the Na^+ gradient across the cell membrane and, as a result, Ca^{2+} is not extruded by the Na^+/Ca^{2+} transporter. This accumulation of Ca^{2+} increases cardiac contractility. At therapeutic doses, cardiac glycosides indirectly decrease heart rate and slow AV conduction by activating parasympathetic vagal nerves. Larger doses can disturb cardiac rhythm because of increased Na^+ and Ca^{2+} levels in myocardial cells. Glycosides and K^+ compete for the Na^+/K^+ ATPace, and loss of extracellular K^+ (e.g. by diuretics) can increase the effectiveness of glycoside, thereby increasing the risk of arrhythmia. At toxic doses, they indirectly increase sympathetic drive, which can increase myocardial excitability, leading to arrhythmias.

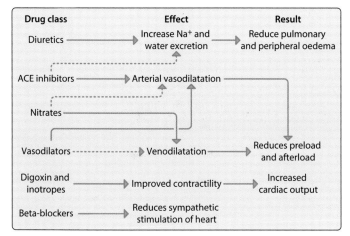

Fig. 3.12.3 Mode of action of drugs used in heart failure.

Phosphodiesterase 3 inhibitors. PDE3 converts cAMP to AMP and so its inhibitors increase intracellular cAMP and augment Ca^{2+} entry into muscle. In cardiac muscle, this increases contractility. PDE3 inhibitors (**milrinone amrinone**) are used in CHF unresponsive to other treatments but worsen survival. Side-effects include nausea, emesis, headache and arrhythmias.

The β_1-adrenoceptor agonists. These (**dobutamine** and **dopamine**) are positive inotropes that are used in emergency situations, acute severe heart failure, as they have been shown to increase mortality.

Preload and/or congestion

Diuretics. Thiazides (**hydrochlorothiazide**, **chlortalidone**) and loop diuretics (**bumetanide**, **furosemide**) reduce venous pressure and cardiac preload, thereby increasing the efficiency of the heart. A major side-effect is reduced K^+ levels, which can cause abnormal heart rhythms when used in combination with glycosides. This can be avoided by using K^+-sparing diuretics (e.g. **spironolactone**, **trimeratene**). (See Ch. 17.)

ACE inhibitors. These drugs (**captopril**, **enalapril**) stimulate dilatation of the arteries and veins, improving cardiac function; reduce cardiac muscle hypertrophy, increasing survival, and promote Na^+ and water loss, thereby reducing congestion. (See Ch. 17.)

Nitrovasodilators. These predominantly work by reducing cardiac preload. **Sodium nitroprusside** has an additional benefit by reducing cardiac afterload. (See Ch. 11.)

Beta-adrenoceptor antagonists

Paradoxically, chronic use of β-adrenoceptor antagonists reduces mortality in CHF. The mechanism may be through antagonism of raised sympathetic drive. These drugs initially reduce heart rate and cardiac output and this may make the patient feel worse; lowering the initial dose will avoid this. As treatment continues, cardiac output is raised and symptoms improve.

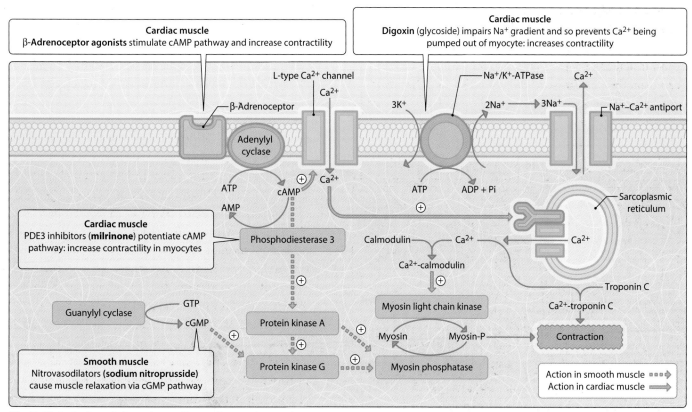

Fig. 3.12.4 Action of drugs in cardiac and smooth muscle.

13. Hypertension

Questions
- How is hypertension defined?
- Why is hypertension dangerous?
- What drugs are used in the treatment of hypertension?

Pathophysiology

Blood pressure is determined by cardiac output, total peripheral resistance and blood volume (Fig. 3.13.1A). Hypertension is defined as a diastolic blood pressure greater than 90–100 mmHg; if untreated, it can be fatal. It can increase the risk of thrombosis, stroke and renal failure. Risk factors for hypertension include obesity, smoking, diabetes, hyperlipidaemia and left ventricular failure, although the underlying cause is not known in the majority (primary or essential hypertension).

Treatment of hypertension

Treatments can be broadly classified according to the primary site of drug action. The pharmacological strategy usually involves combining drug classes and approaches. First line is life style (reduce Na$^+$, alcohol intake, stop smoking) plus diuretics and beta blockers if needed. Mild–moderate hypertension is treated with beta-blocker plus a calcium channel antagonist, or diuretics plus angiotensin-converting enzyme (ACE) inhibitor. Emergency treatment is i.v. sodium nitroprusside.

Diuretics

Diuretics are discussed in Ch. 17. While the initial fall in blood volume correlates with Na$^+$ and water loss, the fall in cardiac output is not maintained despite demonstrable hypotensive action. Furthermore, loop diuretics are only moderately effective antihypertensive agents. Therefore, other mechanisms must account for the reduction of total peripheral resistance with these agents. Thiazide diuretics may activate ATP-dependent potassium channels in resistance arterioles, leading to smooth muscle relaxation. Side-effects of these drugs include hypokalaemia, which can be minimized by using K$^+$ supplements or replacing with K$^+$-sparing diuretic agents. Thiazides may also cause sexual dysfunction in men.

The renin–angiotensin system

ACE inhibitors. These drugs (e.g. **captopril** and **enalapril**) inhibit production of angiotensin II, which is a potent vasoconstrictor both directly and indirectly by stimulating the release of norepinephrine from sympathetic terminals and the secretion of aldosterone from the adrenal cortex (Fig. 3.13.1A). ACE also catalyses the metabolism of bradykinin, a potent vasodilator. Hence, ACE inhibitors reduce total peripheral resistance and blood volume but do not alter cardiac output. Side-effects include cough (caused by increased bradykinin, a known sensitizer of cough receptors).

Angiotensin II inhibitors. The angiotensin II receptor antagonist **losartan** inhibits the peripheral actions of angiotensin II (Fig. 3.13.1B) but does not modify the levels of bradykinin and so does not induce cough.

Spasmolysis

Indirect and direct spasmolytics act via adrenoceptors:

- inhibiting α$_1$-adrenoceptor-mediated blood vessel constriction
- stimulating α$_2$-adrenoceptors centrally and peripherally, inhibiting sympathetic drive
- inhibiting cardiac β$_1$-adrenoceptors, reducing rate and force
- inhibiting β$_2$-adrenoceptors in kidney, promoting water and Na$^+$ exretion.

Beta-blockers. The mechanism of action is not certain but total peripheral resistance falls. The β-adrenoceptor antagonists include **propranolol** (β-non-selective), **atenolol**, **betaxolol**, **bisoprolol** (cardioselective) and **carvedilol**, **labetalol** (α and β non-selective). They may act on the heart to reduce heart rate and contractility, in the kidney to reduce renin secretion and centrally to reduce sympathetic drive to the periphery. Side-effects include cold hands, fatigue and bronchospasm (in asthmatics) and they may be contraindicated in heart block and congestive heart failure (Ch. 11).

Blockers of α$_1$-adrenoceptors. Drugs like **prazosin** and **doxazosin** competitively inhibit α$_1$-adrenoceptors on arteriolar smooth muscle cells, blocking vasoconstriction, thus leading to a fall in total peripheral resistance. Postural hypotension, headache, fatigue, weakness, nausea and palpitations are unwanted side-effects.

Agonists of α$_2$-adrenoceptors. Drugs like **clonidine** and **guanabenz** directly activate presynaptic α$_2$-adrenoceptors, suppressing release of norepinephrine and reducing sympathetic drive to the heart and blood vessels. Adverse effects include sedation, dry mouth and impotence. Rebound hypertension occurs if treatment is withdrawn too quickly.

Calcium channel blockers. The 1,4-dihydropyridines (**nifedipine**, **amlodipine**) block L-type calcium channels on vascular smooth muscle, thereby reducing Ca^{2+} entry and contraction; consequently total peripheral resistance falls. Side-effects include postural hypotension (associated with arteriolar dilatation), dizziness and flushing.

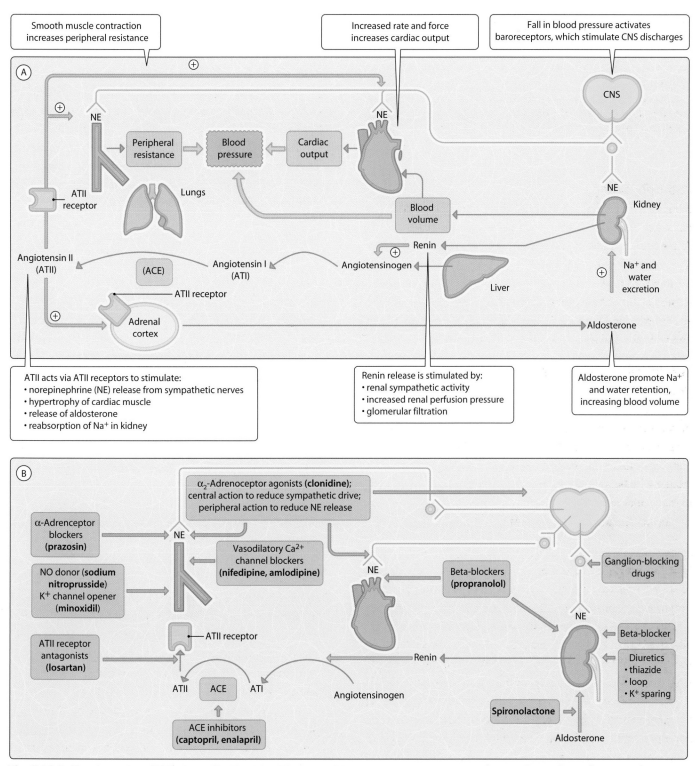

Fig. 3.13.1 Blood pressure. (A) Factors affecting blood pressure; (B) action of antihypertensive drugs. ACE, angiotensin-converting enzyme.

Vasodilators

Drugs that induce vasodilatation and hence reduce total peripheral resistance include **hydralazine** and **sodium nitroprusside** (releases nitric oxide). Side-effects include tachycardia, fluid retention, nausea and vomiting. **Minoxidil** opens ATP-sensitive potassium channels by antagonizing the binding of ATP to the channel (this keeps the channel closed); this results in membrane hyperpolarization, impaired Ca^{2+} entry into vascular smooth muscle cells and spasmolysis. Side-effects include hirsutism (in women), tachycardia, Na^+ and water retention and cardiotoxicity.

14. Haemostasis and thrombosis

Questions
- What factors regulate haemostasis?
- What drugs are used in the treatment and prevention of thrombosis?

Haemostasis

The body responds to a rupture of the blood vessels by constriction, platelet aggregation, plug formation and blood clotting. Disruption of blood vessels exposes underlying collagen, which platelets adhere to by binding von Willebrand factor (vWF). This results in platelet activation and release of vasoconstrictors such as thromboxane A_2, thereby reducing blood flow to the affected area. This mediator, along with platelet-derived ADP, serotonin and thrombin (factor IIa), causes other platelets to aggregate. The surrounding undamaged endothelium releases prostaglandin I_2 (prostacyclin) and nitric oxide, which serve to limit platelet adherence and aggregation. The activation of thrombin converts soluble fibrinogen to fibrin. Liquid blood is converted to a solid gel reinforcing the platelet plug, which consists of aggregating platelets, fibrin and trapped red blood cells. The pathological formation of a clot can cause occlusion within blood vessels, leading to myocardial infarction, stroke and peripheral ischaemia (arterial side), deep vein thrombosis (DVT) and pulmonary embolism (venous side) and death.

Treatment of thrombosis

Drugs used in the treatment of thrombosis interfere with the coagulation pathway (Fig. 3.14.1), platelets (Fig. 3.14.2) or the fibrinolytic pathway (Fig. 3.14.1) and are generally used in combination for optimal results (Fig. 3.14.3).

Anticoagulants

Warfarin. Thrombin plays a central role in haemostasis and acts in a positive feedback loop to stimulate its own formation. Several coagulation factors, including factors II, VII, IX and X, require post-transcriptional carboxylation of their glutamic acid residues for full enzymatic activity and are dependent upon the oxidation of vitamin K, an essential cofactor in this process. Warfarin inhibits vitamin K epoxide reductase, a hepatic enzyme (Fig. 3.14.2). A delay (approximately 5 days) in the anticoagulant action of warfarin is observed because of slow clearance of existing γ-carboxylated coagulation factors from the circulation (prothrombin has the longest elimination half-life). Warfarin is administered orally; side-effects include haemorrhage and teratogenicity (avoided in the first trimester).

Heparin. Heparin is a negatively charged glycosaminoglycan of varying molecular weight (5–30 kDa). It potentiates the action of antithrombin III, which inhibits thrombin and other serine proteases including coagulation factors XIIa, XIa, IXa and Xa (Fig. 3.14.1). Heparin induces a conformational change in antithrombin III, making the reactive site more accessible to proteases. Heparin (unfractionated) infusion or s.c. injections reduce the incidence of DVT in patients undergoing surgery or recovering from strokes and myocardial infarctions; it also prevents clotting in catheters. Treatment with heparin can cause bleeding but this can be controlled as the half-life is short (4–6 h) and its effect can be reduced by injection with **protamine**, a positively charged basic peptide. Thrombocytopenia can also be an unwanted side-effect, and subjects should be monitored closely. **Low-molecular-weight heparins** (< 18 kDa) offer

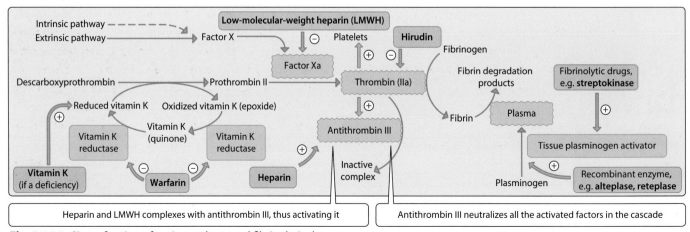

Heparin and LMWH complexes with antithrombin III, thus activating it

Antithrombin III neutralizes all the activated factors in the cascade

Fig. 3.14.1 Sites of action of anticoagulants and fibrinolytic drugs.

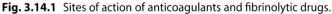

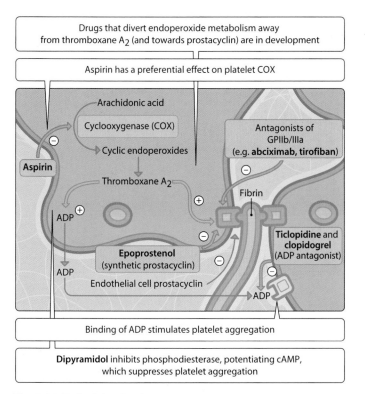

Fig. 3.14.2 Antiplatelet drugs.

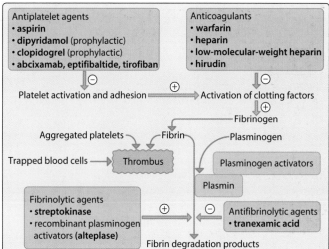

Fig. 3.14.3 Coordinated strategy in thrombosis.

the advantage of greater duration of action, better bioavailability and appear to have a greater selective inhibitory action for factor IXa.

Antiplatelet agents

Aspirin. Aspirin is a non-selective cyclooxygenase (COX) inhibitor, reducing the formation of platelet-derived thromboxane A₂ (Fig. 3.14.2). Aspirin is used prophylactically to reduce the incidence of myocardial infarction, risk of stroke and coronary thrombosis. Side-effects include gastric bleeding, ulceration with overdose, reduced renal function owing to reduced renal blood flow and, occasionally, bronchospasm in asthma.

ADP antagonists. Drugs like **ticlopidine** and **clopidogrel** inhibit binding of ADP to the platelet receptor (Fig. 3.14.2). ADP released from activated platelets induces the expression of glycoprotein (GP) IIb/IIIa receptor, which binds fibrinogen. ADP antagonists also interfere with binding of vWF to platelet GPIB receptors. Thus, platelet adhesion and aggregation are inhibited. These drugs have a synergistic action when used in combination with aspirin or

GPIIb/IIIa receptor antagonists. Adverse effects include gastrointestinal bleeding and, in rare cases, neutropenia and agranulocytosis.

Glycoprotein IIb/IIIa receptor antagonists. Fibrinogen binding to platelet cell surface GPIIb/IIIa receptors allows adjacent platelets to adhere and provides additional binding for vWF and fibronectin (Fig. 3.14.2). The monoclonal antibody **abciximab** and synthetic agents like **eptifibatide** and **tirofiban** inhibit binding of fibrinogen and other adhesive proteins to GPIIb/IIIa. These agents are administered i.v. and bleeding is a side-effect.

Dipyramidol. This is used in combination with warfarin to prevent thrombosis in patients with prosthetic heart valves. It inhibits phosphodiesterase, thus raising cAMP in platelets and reducing platelet aggregation (Fig. 3.14.2). Side-effects include nausea, diarrhoea, hypotension and headache.

Fibrinolytic agents

Plasminogen is an endogenous activator of plasmin, a protein that degrades fibrin and plays an important role in clot resolution (Fig. 3.14.3). Fibrinolytic agents like **streptokinase** and human tissue plasmin activators (tpA, **alteplase**) activate plasminogen to form plasmin. These drugs are administered i.v. in life-threatening venous thrombosis, pulmonary embolism, arterial thromboembolism and acute myocardial infarction. To be optimally effective, fibrinolytic agents should be given within 90 min of infarction.

15. Dyslipidaemia and lipid-lowering drugs

Questions
- Why are dyslipidaemias a health risk?
- What drugs are used in the treatment of dyslipidaemia?

Physiology of lipoproteins

The metabolism of lipoproteins is complex (Fig. 3.15.1) and alterations in lipid metabolism can result in dyslipidaemias characterized by elevated levels of low density lipoprotein (LDL) and reduced levels of high density lipoprotein (HDL). Physiologically, HDL plays a 'protective' role against atherosclerotic disease in the sense that it lacks class B and E lipoproteins needed for LDL particle uptake by extrahepatic tissue and it has a role in 'reverse cholesterol transport' from extrahepatic tissue to the liver. Alterations in the levels of lipoproteins predispose individuals to the formation of atherosclerotic plaques, resulting in coronary artery disease. A variety of factors including a poor diet, lack of exercise and genetic predisposition (e.g. type IIa dyslipidaemia or familial hypercholesterolaemia caused by a defect in the LDL receptor) result in high plasma cholesterol levels and cardiovascular disease.

Treatment of high cholesterol and triacylglycerols

There are three major drug classes used to reduce circulating cholesterol and triacylglycerols (triglycerides): those that inhibit cholesterol absorption (bile acid-binding resins), those reducing its synthesis (statins) and those promoting its metabolism (fibrates) (Fig. 3.15.2).

Bile acid-binding resins

Bile acids excreted in the gastrointestinal tract promote the absorption of dietary fat. Binding resins interfere with this process by forming complexes with bile acids. Binding resins like **colestyramine**, **colestipol** and **colesevelam** are ingested orally and are not absorbed from the gastrointestinal tract. Two important consequences arise from the inactivation of bile acids in the gastrointestinal tract. First, the absorption of cholesterol and triacylglycerols is impaired and, second, the enterohepatic reabsorption of bile acids is broken. The liver responds by diverting de novo synthesized cholesterol to bile acids and increases the expression of LDL receptors to facilitate cholesterol uptake by the liver. As a result, plasma LDL levels fall and a mild-to-moderate reduction in plasma cholesterol levels ensues. These drugs are effective in type II hypercholesterolaemia and

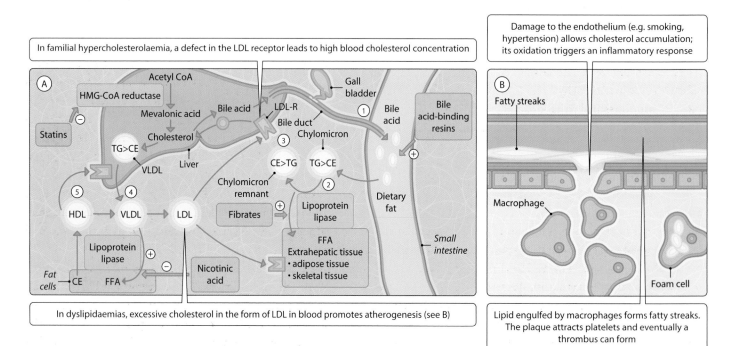

Fig. 3.15.1 Metabolism of lipoproteins. 1. Cholesterol and free fatty acids (FFA) are absorbed from the small intestine with the aid of bile acids and form chylomicrons. 2. Lipoprotein lipase on the capillary epithelium of skeletal muscle and adipocytes removes FFAs. 3. The chylomicron remnant is absorbed by the liver via the low density lipoprotein (LDL) receptor and cholesterol is utilized in the formation of bile acids and steroid precursors. 4. Surplus cholesterol is transported to peripheral cells as very low density lipoproteins (VLDL). 5. Cholesterol is carried away from the tissues to the liver as high density lipoproteins (HDL).

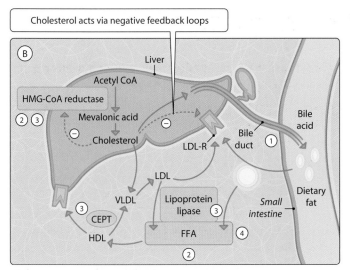

Fig. 3.15.2 Treatment of hypercholesterolaemia. 1. Bile acid-binding resins reduce enterohepatic recycling of bile acids, leading to a compensatory increase in bile acid synthesis from cholesterol. The negative feedback effect of cholesterol on HMG-CoA reductase and on expression of LDL receptor is reduced and leads to increased uptake of LDL from plasma. 2. Statins are competitive reversible inhibitors of HMG-CoA reductase and so reduce cholesterol synthesis in the liver. This again reduces plasma LDL. They also have other useful non-lipid roles (see text). 3. Fibrates modify the transcription of genes involved in lipid metabolism, increasing the activity of lipoprotein lipase in extrahepatic tissue, promoting uptake of triacylglycerol-rich VLDL and chylomicrons into target tissues, thereby reducing plasma triacylglycerols, and reducing VLDL synthesis in the liver. 4. Nicotinic acid inhibits hormone-sensitive lipase in adipose tissue, reduces triacylglycerol synthesis in the liver and formation of VLDL. CEPT, cholesteryl ester transfer protein.

reduce the incidence of coronary artery disease, but they are not effective alone in familial hypercholesterolaemia. Adverse effects include gastrointestinal irritation, and patient compliance is an issue because these drugs must be consumed three times daily. The drugs also interfere with the absorption of drugs such as warfarin and digoxin and therefore should not be taken together.

Statins

The rate-limiting step in the synthesis of cholesterol by the liver is the conversion of 3-hydroxy-3-methylglutaryl (HMG)-CoA to mevalonate by the enzyme HMG-CoA reductase. Statins (e.g. **simvastatin**, **atorvastatin**, **lovastatin**) are competitive inhibitors of this enzyme, reducing the availability of cholesterol for bile acids and resulting in a fall in lipid absorption from the gastrointestinal tract. Furthermore, the body compensates for the disruption in cholesterol synthesis by increasing the expression of LDL receptor, which increases the clearance of LDL and reduces cholesterol in the plasma. Since LDL is cleared from the plasma, triacylglycerols will also fall. Statins have other

relevant actions: they improve endothelial cell function, stabilize the atherosclerotic plaque, reduce platelet aggregation, enhance fibrinolysis and reduce inflammatory cell recruitment into plaques. These drugs produce a mild-to-moderate reduction in plasma cholesterol in type II hypercholesterolaemia and reduce the incidence of coronary artery disease. Constipation, diarrhoea, nausea, headache, fatigue or insomnia are reported side-effects. A rare adverse event is a reversible myositis.

Fibrates

Fibrates (e.g. **ciprofibrate**, **gemfibrozil**, **clofibrate** and **fenofibrate**) have a predominant action on very low density lipoproteins (VLDL) rather than LDL. It has recently been shown that these drugs can modify the transcription of a variety of genes involved in lipid metabolism via activation of peroxisomal proliferator-activated receptors (PPAR). This increases the activity of lipoprotein lipase in extrahepatic tissue (e.g. skeletal muscle, fat cells) and promotes the hydrolysis of triacylglycerol-rich VLDL and chylomicrons to facilitate uptake into target tissues, thereby reducing plasma triacylglycerols. These drugs also reduce the synthesis of VLDL in the liver and the remnants are diverted to the synthesis of HDL. These drugs produce variable (small) falls in plasma LDL. They also increase fatty acid breakdown and inhibit fatty acid synthesis. These drugs are used in types IIb, III and V hyperlipidaemia and for prevention of coronary artery disease. Side-effects include myositis-like syndrome, gastrointestinal disturbances, headache, blurred vision, dizziness and rash.

Other drugs

Nicotinic acid.   Niacin (nicotinic acid) is a vitamin precursor of nicotine adenine dinucleotides but suppresses lipolysis of triacylglycerols in adipose tissue independently of this activity. Nicotinic acid inhibits the activity of hormone-sensitive lipase in adipose tissue and reduces triacylglycerol synthesis in the liver and formation of VLDL. This fall in VLDL also leads to an increase in HDL since the plasma transfer of cholesteryl esters from HDL to VLDL is reduced. This drug can be used for type IIb hyperlipidaemia; its side-effects include flushing, headache, palpitation, nausea and vomiting.

Probucol.   Oxidation of LDL promotes its accumulation in atherosclerotic lesions and phagocytosis by macrophages. Probucol has antioxidant activity that accounts for its anti-atherogenic activity. Paradoxically, probucol enhances the activity of cholesteryl-ester transfer protein, which promotes the movement of cholesteryl esters from HDL to VLDL and thereby reduces plasma HDL. It, therefore, has limited utility and is also associated with ventricular arrhythmias.

16. Agents used in the treatment of anaemia

Questions
- What are the important features of anaemia?
- What drugs are used in the treatment of anaemia?

Normal red blood cell (RBC) production requires erythropoietin, vitamin B_{12} (cobalamin), folic acid and iron (Fig. 3.16.1) and deficiency in any of these cofactors can cause anaemia. Symptoms reflect a decrease in the oxygen-carrying capacity of red blood cells and include pallor, shortness of breath and fatigue.

Treatment of anaemias
Hypoproliferative (low RBC production) anaemias are treated by supplementation with iron, vitamin B_{12}, folates and **epoetin** (recombinant erythropoietin). Hyperproliferative (increased peripheral destruction of RBC) anaemias (e.g. sickle cell anaemia) are treated with **hydroxyurea**, which increases haemoglobin F production.

Iron supplements. A common cause of anaemia is iron deficiency in chronic blood loss (menstruation), in pregnancy and in pathological blood loss (e.g. from gastrointestinal bleeding). Diagnostically, RBCs appear small (microcytosis). Treatment with iron supplements (ferrous sulphate, oral) may cause gastrointestinal irritation in some subjects, which can be minimized by ingestion with food. Parenteral administration (i.v.) is required for those with chronic bleeding disorders and, therefore, cannot tolerate oral administration. In certain circumstances, iron toxicity can be fatal, particularly in children who inadvertently overdose on iron supplements or in individuals with β-thalassaemia and who require regular blood transfusions (iron load is increased). The body does not have a mechanism to excrete excess iron but iron levels can be corrected with the use of selective iron chelators such as **desferrioxamine** (Fig. 3.16.1).

Vitamin B_{12}. Vitamin B_{12} comprises a cobalt atom attached to four pyrrole rings and a nucleoside; it is absorbed from the diet in a complex with intrinsic factor (Fig. 3.16.2). Vitamin B_{12} is an important cofactor in enzyme reactions required for the synthesis of DNA and biochemical defects here result in megaloblastic anaemia. Cell types with high rates of DNA synthesis are susceptible to vitamin B_{12} deficiency (Fig. 3.16.2B).

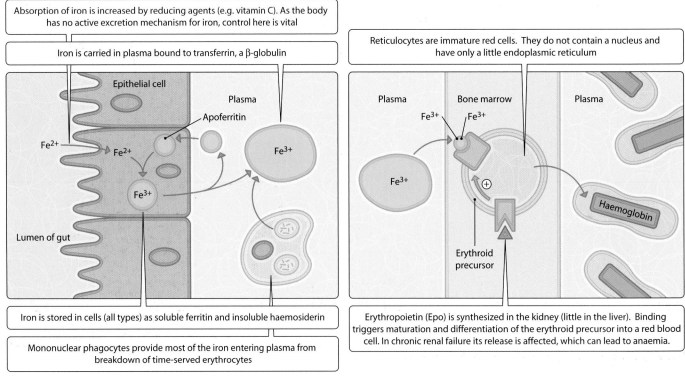

Fig. 3.16.1 Red blood cell production.

Diagnosis of vitamin B_{12} deficiency involves measuring its serum levels (will fall) and methylmalonic acid (will rise). The Schilling test is used for pernicious anaemia. Intramuscular injection may be required in pernicious anaemia since oral bioavailability will be poor. Supplementation with folic acid will reverse anaemia but will not alter any neurological deficits.

Folic acid. Dietary folates (fresh green vegetables, liver, yeast, fruits) are polyglutamates that are hydrolysed to mono- and diglutamates before being absorbed from the gut. Folic acid as N^5-methyltetrahydrofolic acid is stored in the liver and rapidly transported to tissues bound to plasma proteins. It is transported into rapidly dividing cells where it undergoes conversion to tetrahydrofolate by a vitamin B_{12}-dependent process. Tetrahydrofolate is an important cofactor, donating a one-carbon atom unit in the synthesis of thymidylic acid, an important precursor of DNA. Folic acid deficiencies may arise in chronic alcoholism, inflammatory bowel disease, coeliac sprue, when demand is high (e.g. in pregnancy) or as a consequence of treatment with methotrexate (antifolate). Macrocytosis and folate deficiency in plasma diagnose this deficiency. It is important to exclude vitamin B_{12} deficiency since supplementation with folic acid alone will not correct the associated neurological deficits.

Epoetin. Erythropoietin is an endogenous growth factor released from the kidney in response to hypoxia and is critical in the differentiation of erythroid progenitor cells to RBCs. Epoetin is administered s.c. or i.v. in patients with renal failure and significant anaemia. It is also indicated in primary bone marrow disorders and secondary anaemia associated with inflammation, AIDS and cancer. It is banned by the International Olympic Committee.

Hyperproliferative anaemia. Anaemias associated with increased production and destruction of RBCs result in hyperproliferative anaemias. Sickle cell anaemia is a common haemoglobinopathy. A point mutation in the gene transcribing the β-chain of haemoglobin S (valine at position 6 to glutamate) results in polymerization of haemoglobin S and deformity of RBC (sickling) and haemolysis. Microvascular occlusion is a characteristic of this disease.

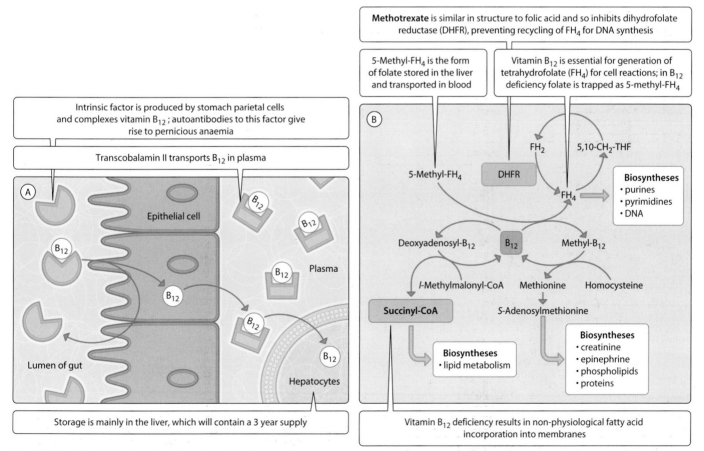

Fig. 3.16.2 Vitamin B_{12} uptake (A) and metabolic role (B).

17. Diuretics

Questions
- How are body fluids regulated?
- What drugs are used to alter body fluid?

The kidney is the site of excretion of metabolic waste and drugs; it regulates body water and mineral content and secretes hormones (renin, erythropoietin) (Fig. 3.17.1). Any condition that leads to an increase in interstitial (extracellular) volume (e.g. nephrotic syndrome, liver disease and congestive heart failure) will result in tissue swelling and symptoms (e.g. dyspnoea in pulmonary oedema). In nephrotic syndrome, there is an increase in the permeability of the glomerular basement membrane to proteins, leading to a marked loss of protein in the urine (proteinuria). This loss of protein results in a fall in plasma protein oncotic (colloidal) pressure and, hence, fluid flows into the extracellular spaces. This fall in blood volume then activates the renin–angiotensin system to promote Na^+ and water retention by the kidneys, thereby increasing fluid retention by tissues. In liver disease, a decrease in protein synthesis also reduces hydrostatic pressure within the circulation, which favours the flow of water into tissues (e.g. peritoneal cavity; a process termed ascites). The ensuing loss in blood volume activates the renin–angiotensin system.

Drug treatment

A variety of drugs promote Na^+ excretion and water loss by a selective action on the kidney (Fig. 3.17.1).

Carbonic anhydrase inhibitors

In the proximal tubule, 60% of filtered Na^+ reabsorption is driven by Na^+/K^+-ATPase. However, some active transport of Na^+ is dependent upon the activity of carbonic anhydrase, an enzyme important for the reabsorption of bicarbonate ions. Carbonic anhydrase inhibitors (**acetazolamide**) disrupt the formation of carbonic acid and diminish the reabsorption of bicarbonate and consequently Na^+ via the Na^+/H^+ antiport. The increase in luminal Na^+ load is easily reabsorbed in the thick ascending limb of the nephron and, therefore, there is only a modest increase in Na^+ excretion and water loss. This drug is mainly used in the treatment of glaucoma to reduce aqueous humour formation.

Osmotic diuretics

Osmotic diuretics increase the osmolarity of the glomerular filtrate, thereby preventing water reabsorption by the kidney. These drugs are not completely absorbed from the lumen of the nephron and so increase luminal osmolarity. Water is normally free to move out of the proximal tubule, descending limb of the loop of Henle and collecting duct to be reabsorbed, but the

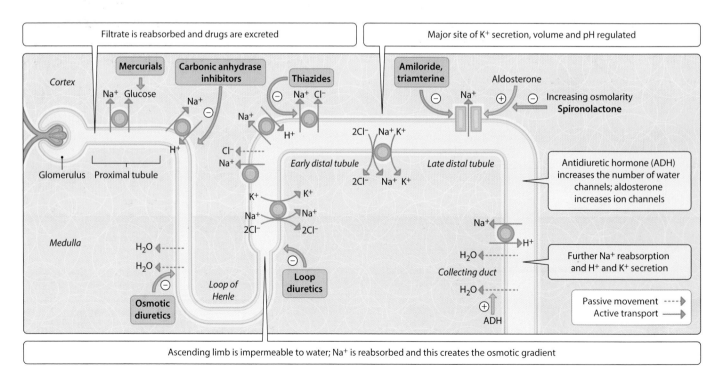

Fig. 3.17.1 Drugs acting on the kidney.

increased osmolarity preferentially retains it in the lumen for excretion. An increase in blood osmolarity also increases blood volume through the net movement of water from extracellular spaces to the blood compartment; this increase in blood volume impairs renin release from the kidney, which also promotes loss of Na^+ and water. These agents may be used in acute renal failure to promote renal blood flow and diuresis and are administered i.v. (**mannitol**) or orally (**glycerin, isosorbide**).

Loop diuretics

The ascending limb of the loop of Henle is an important site that enables the kidney to establish an osmotic gradient for the reabsorption of water from the collecting tubule. Loop diuretics (**furosemide, bumetanide**) inhibit the co-transporter for Na^+, K^+ and Cl^- on the apical surface of tubular epithelial cells in the thick ascending limb of the loop of Henle. These drugs are highly efficacious and commonly referred to as high-ceiling diuretics, as they prevent the reabsorption of Na^+ and, by reducing the osmotic gradient within the medulla, impair water reabsorption from the collecting duct. The increase in luminal Na^+ load that reaches the late distal tubules drives K^+ excretion, resulting in hypokalaemia. These drugs are used in acute pulmonary oedema, nephrotic syndrome and hypertension. Adverse effects include hypokalaemia (corrected with potassium ion supplementation), Ca^{2+} and Mg^{2+} deficiency, metabolic alkalosis, hypovolaemia and hypotension.

Thiazide diuretics

Thiazide (**hydrochlorothiazide, polythiazide, indapamide, chlortalidone, metolazone**) act by blocking the Na^+/Cl^- symporter on the apical membrane of epithelial cells in the distal tubule. These drugs have a moderate diuretic effect as most of the Na^+ has been reabsorbed prior to entering the distal tubules. Like loop diuretics, they promote the excretion of K^+ into the collecting ducts but, unlike loop diuretics, they reduce Ca^{2+} excretion. Thiazide diuretics cause hypokalaemia and acidosis. These drugs are used for hypertension, oedema caused by congestive heart failure, liver disease or nephrotic syndrome.

Potassium-sparing diuretics

Sodium channel blockers. Sodium channels (different to voltage-gated sodium channels) facilitate the movement of Na^+ across the apical membrane. The electrochemical gradient generated by the Na^+/K^+-ATPase on the basolateral membrane drives Na^+ entry, which generates an important negative driving force for the efflux of K^+ into the lumen. This negative driving force also explains why carbonic anhydrase inhibitors, loop diuretics and thiazides promote K^+ secretion, as they increase Na^+ burden to the distal tubules. Sodium channel blockers (e.g. **amiloride, triamterene**) promote Na^+ excretion while K^+ excretion is inhibited; they are K^+ sparing.

Aldosterone antagonists. Aldosterone promotes the activity of a variety of transporters and pumps involved in the absorption of Na^+. This hormone increases the transcription of proteins, which activates silent (non-functional) sodium channels, increases the synthesis of Na^+/K^+-ATPase, Na^+/H^+-antiport, potassium channels, H^+/ATPase and mitochondrial synthesis of ATP. The net effect is to enhance NaCl absorption. Aldosterone inhibitors like **spironolactone** bind to the aldosterone receptor in tubule epithelial cells but do not lead to gene transcription. This class also has K^+-sparing activities. Adverse effects result from non-specific binding to other steroid receptors and include gynaecomastia, menstrual disorders, impotence and loss of libido.

18. Gastrointestinal tract: anti-ulcer agents

Questions
- How are gastrointestinal ulcers formed?
- What drugs are used in their treatment?

The gastrointestinal tract is principally concerned with the breakdown of food and absorption of amino acids, peptides, carbohydrates, sugars and lipids. These are transported to the liver for conversion into proteins, carbohydrates and lipids for the body's needs. The digestion of food involves the release of gastric acid from parietal cells of the stomach, digestive enzymes and mucus (Fig. 3.18.1). An imbalance between acid production and the mucus barrier protecting the epithelium lead to tissue damage through the corrosive action of gastric acid, resulting in peptic ulcers (in stomach (gastric) and duodenum). Peptic ulcers are characterized by mucosal bleeding, perforation and, when situated near the pyloric sphincter, obstruction of food leaving the stomach. Symptoms of peptic ulcers include burning sensation below the breastbone, nausea, vomiting and, in more severe cases, persistent stomach pain, bloody or black stools and bloody vomit. Causative factors include *Helicobacter pylori* infection, chronic use of NSAIDs, genetic factors, alcohol and stress. A variety of treatment strategies exist for peptic ulcers and include eradication of *H. pylori* infection (antibiotics), inhibition of acid secretion (histamine H_2 antagonists, proton pump inhibitors (PPIs)), cytoprotective agents and mucosal strengtheners (prostaglandins, antacids, sucralfate) (Fig. 3.18.2).

Helicobacter pylori infection

H. pylori infection is a predominant predisposing factor for gastric ulcers, and treatment with a cocktail of antibiotics can significantly reduce the incidence of this disease. The current recommendation is triple therapy with two antibiotics (**clarythromycin** plus either **metronidazole** or **amoxicillin**) and a PPI.

Antisecretory agents

Proton pump inhibitors. The PPIs (**omeprazole, lansopranzole, rabeprazole, esomeprazole, pantoprazole**) cause irreversible inhibition of H^+/K^+-ATPase and inhibit acid secretion promoted by various stimuli including acetylcholine, histamine and gastrin (Fig. 3.18.2). PPIs are inactive prodrugs converted to sulphonamides in the acidic environment of the secretory canaliculi of parietal cells; they covalently bind to SH groups on H^+/K^+-ATPase. The active metabolite does not readily cross cell membranes and, therefore, has little action on other ion pumps within the body. These drugs are highly effective, resulting in 90% inhibition of acid production throughout a 24 h period. Side-effects include headache, skin rashes and gastrointestinal upset. PPIs (e.g. omeprazole) inhibit cytochrome P450 and, therefore, should be avoided in subjects taking warfarin, theophylline and phenytoin.

Histamine H_2 receptor antagonists. Histamine stimulates gastric acid secretion via H_2 receptors on parietal cells (Fig. 3.18.2). A number of potent H_2 receptor antagonists include **cimetidine, ranitidine, famotidine** and **nizatidine**. These drugs are less effective than the PPIs since gastric acid secretion is also stimulated following activation of muscarinic and gastrin receptors on parietal cells. These drugs relieve the pain of ulcers, promote healing and are administered at night time when acid buffering is at its lowest. The usual regimen is twice daily treatment for 4–8 weeks. Cimetidine inhibits cytochrome P450 and should be avoided by patients taking warfarin, phenytoin and theophylline.

Anticholinergic drugs. **Pirenzepine** is a competitive antagonist at muscarinic M_1 receptors on parasympathetic ganglia and, to a lesser extent, on M_2 receptors present on parietal cells (Fig. 3.18.2). These agents reduce gastric acid secretion via vagal stimulation. Pirenzepine is not the drug of first choice since gastric acid secretion can be induced by gastrin and histamine. Absorption of pirenzepine from the gut is poor and it does not cross the blood–brain barrier. Side-effects include dry mouth and blurred vision.

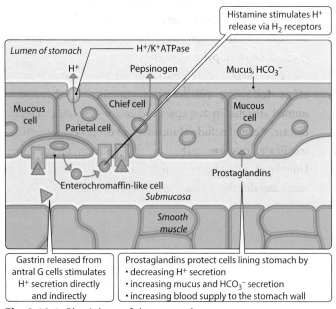

Fig. 3.18.1 Physiology of the stomach.

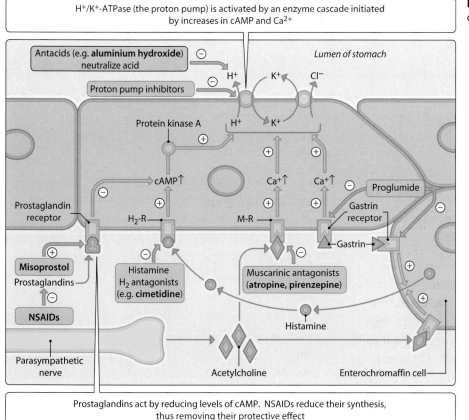

Fig. 3.18.2 Acid secretion from parietal cells and the sites of drug action.

Within the figure:

H$^+$/K$^+$-ATPase (the proton pump) is activated by an enzyme cascade initiated by increases in cAMP and Ca^{2+}

Antacids (e.g. **aluminium hydroxide**) neutralize acid

Lumen of stomach

Proton pump inhibitors

H$^+$ K$^+$ Cl$^-$

Protein kinase A H$^+$ K$^+$

cAMP↑ Ca$^+$↑ Ca$^+$↑ Proglumide

Prostaglandin receptor H$_2$-R M-R Gastrin receptor

Gastrin

Misoprostol Histamine H$_2$ antagonists (e.g. **cimetidine**) Muscarinic antagonists (**atropine, pirenzepine**)

Prostaglandins

NSAIDs Histamine

Parasympathetic nerve Acetylcholine Enterochromaffin cell

Prostaglandins act by reducing levels of cAMP. NSAIDs reduce their synthesis, thus removing their protective effect

Cytoprotective agents and mucosal strengtheners

Prostaglandins. Endogenous prostanoids like prostaglandin E$_2$ and prostaglandin I$_2$ (prostacyclin) are cytoprotective. The prostaglandin analogue **misoprostol** is a protective agent that inhibits acid secretion, promotes bicarbonate formation and mucus secretion, and increases blood flow; consequently, it promotes ulcer healing and is co-prescribed in subjects who are taking NSAIDs over prolonged periods, being used as a preventative measure. Side-effects include diarrhoea and abdominal cramps, and it should be avoided in pregnancy. Menorrhagia and postmenopausal bleeding may occur.

Sucralfate. Sucralfate is an aluminium salt of sucrose octasulphate that polymerizes to form a gel in the acid environment of the gut; this gel binds mucosal glyco-proteins in the ulcer crater and forms a protective physical barrier to acid and pepsin. It may also stimulate the production of cytoprotective prostanoids and bicarbonate. Sucralfate also reduces the number of *H. pylori* and its adherence to gastric mucosa, which might explain the lower recurrence rate with its usage. While sucralfate is poorly absorbed, it can induce renal impairment in some individuals and it also causes constipation.

Bismuth chelate. Has similar actions to sucralfate and is used in triple therapy regiment for treating peptic ulcers for eradication of *H. pylori* infection.

Antacids. These agents neutralize acid and have a better effect following consumption of food and provide immediate relief in dyspepsia and gastro-oesophageal reflux disease. Agents include **aluminium hydroxide**, **magnesium trisilicate**, **calcium carbonate** and **sodium bicarbonate**. Unwanted side-effects include constipation (aluminium salts) and diarrhoea (magnesium salts).

19. Gastrointestinal tract: motility and secretions

Questions
- How is gastrointestinal motility controlled?
- What drugs are used for the treatment of gastric motility disorders?

The efficient movement of digested food, nutrients and waste is dependent upon a balance of absorption and secretion of water and electrolytes by the intestine. The movement of contents within the intestine is caused by the peristaltic action of the smooth muscles, which is controlled by the enteric nervous system and various hormones and neurotransmitters (Fig. 3.19.1). Any alteration in intestinal motility can give rise to constipation or diarrhoea and is a feature of irritable bowel syndrome and inflammatory bowel disease.

Constipation
Laxatives promoting defecation include:

- **bulking agents** (e.g. bran, methylcellulose): increase bulk matter within the lumen, thereby stimulating stretch receptors in the intestinal wall and indirectly stimulating muscle contractility
- **water-retaining agents**: saline (e.g. **Epsom salts**) and osmotic agents (**lactulose**) are poorly absorbed from the gastrointestinal tract and lead to retention of water within the lumen by osmosis, thereby facilitating bulk mass and transit
- **stimulant (irritant) laxatives** (e.g. **Senna**, **bisacodyl**, **phenolphthalein**): promote water and electrolyte accumulation in the colon and stimulate muscle motility by stimulating the enteric nervous system
- **faecal softeners** (e.g. docusate) or **lubricants** (e.g. liquid paraffin): improve transit of contents within the colon (Fig. 3.19.1).

Increasing water and fibre content in the diet will also improve transit time within the gastrointestinal tract.

Prokinetic (motility-promoting) drugs
Agents that increase muscle motility of the gastrointestinal tract (prokinetic) but without laxative actions are used in a number of motility disorders, including gastrointestinal reflux and gastric stasis, where increased gastric emptying is desirable. **Domperidone** and **metoclopromide** are dopamine D_2 antagonists used in the treatment of nausea and emesis (Ch. 20). Domperidone also increases gastric motility by a poorly defined mechanism and metoclopromide possibly acts on serotonin

$5HT_4$ receptors on gastrointestinal intrinsic neurons to increase acetylcholine release, thereby increasing motility and gastric emptying. **Cisapride** also stimulates acetylcholine release from intrinsic neurons in the myenteric plexus via a $5HT_4$ receptor-dependent mechanism, thereby promoting gastric motility. Domperidone does not cross the blood–brain barrier and so is preferable to metoclopromide.

Antidiarrhoeal drugs
Diarrhoea is the frequent passage of stools, occurring in gastrointestinal infections, exposure to toxins, drugs, anxiety and chronic disease. The aim of treatment is to promote rehydration, which can be achieved by replenishment with fluid and electrolytes, and treatment of excessive bowel movement. Bulking agents like **kaolin** (absorbent clay) improve stool consistency. Other bulking agents include **wheat bran**, which increases stool viscosity. Treatment with antibiotics should only be used for specific bacterial infections. Drug therapy for diarrhoea includes opioid agonists (e.g. **codeine**, **diphenoxylate**, **loperamide**). Loperamide does not penetrate the blood–brain barrier and so unwanted central side-effects are minimized. These drugs bind to opioid μ receptors on enteric neurons leading to hyperpolarization and reduction of acetylcholine release, resulting in a reduction in peristaltic activity and secretions.

Irritable bowel syndrome
Irritable bowel syndrome is a common intestinal disorder that affects the large intestine and is characterized by abdominal discomfort (e.g. pain, variable bowel movement, bloating). Treatment usually involves antispasmodic agents, including muscarinic antagonists (e.g. **atropine**, **propantheline**), which induce smooth muscle relaxation by indirectly preventing the spasmogenic actions of acetylcholine. Direct-acting spasmolytic agents include **mebeverine**, **alverine** and **peppermint oil** and are used to relieve pain in irritable bowel syndrome.

Inflammatory bowel disease
Inflammatory bowel disease is a chronic inflammatory disorder of the gastrointestinal tract and includes ulcerative colitis and Crohn's disease. The former only affects the large intestine (e.g. colon and rectum) but Crohn's disease affects any part of the tract. Symptoms include abdominal pain, diarrhoea, rectal bleeding, fever, weight loss and anaemia. Treatment entails the use of anti-inflammatory and immunosuppressant drugs. NSAIDs should be avoided. Drugs need to be delivered in an active state to the lower intestine and various methods are used to achieve this.

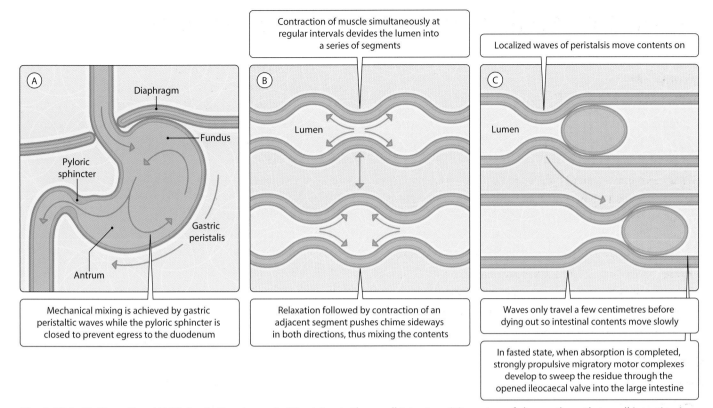

Fig. 3.19.1 Motile action. (A) Mixing in the stomach; (B) mixing in the small intestine: (C) moving of chyme along the small intestine (peristalsis).

Anti-inflammatory drugs. **Sulfasalazine** has the active aspirin-like compound 5-aminosalicylate linked to sulfapyridine; the 5-aminosalicylate is released by bacterial metabolism in the terminal ileum and colon. Sulfapyridine is responsible for the adverse reactions, including nausea and toxic effects on red blood cells. Newer agents avoid the sulfapyridine moiety to achieve a lower side-effect profile. **Mesalamine** lacks the sulfapyridine moiety and oral formulations use coatings or time-released formulations to avoid drug absorption from the upper intestine. **Olsalazine** is two molecules of 5-aminosalicylate linked by a diazo bond, which is cleaved by bacteria in the colon. **Glucocorticosteroids** are widely used to treat relapse and have anti-inflammatory activity. Their oral bioavailability accounts for adverse effects on the endocrine system. **Budesonide** is poorly absorbed from the gastrointestinal tract and has a better tolerability profile.

Immunosuppressant drugs. These drugs are used to suppress the activity of the immune system; **azathioprine**, **6-mercaptopurine**, and **methotrexate** are commonly used. **Infliximab** is a monoclonal antibody against tumour necrosis factor alpha that can induce remission for several months in Crohn's disease.

Antibiotics. Although no specific infectious agent has been found as a causative agent for inflammatory bowel disease, antibiotics, commonly **metronidazole** and **ciprofloxacin**, are used.

Pancreatic supplements

Enzymes important for the breakdown of proteins (trypsin, chymotrypsin), starch (amylase) and fats (lipase) are secreted by the pancreas. **Pancreatin** is an extract containing these enzymes and is administered orally to compensate for reduced or absent secretion by the pancreas in cystic fibrosis, following pancreatectomy and in chronic pancreatitis. Gastric acid inactivates these enzymes, which can be minimized by prior treatment with a histamine H_2 blocker or by using acid-resistant formulations.

Gallstones

Bile (cholesterol, phospholipids and bile salts) is synthesized in the liver and stored in the gall bladder. Bile salts are necessary for absorption of fats from the intestine. Gallstones of precipitated cholesterol occur in inflammation of the gall bladder (cholecystitis) and can be dissolved by drug therapy; however, in most cases surgery is the preferred option. Prolonged treatment with **ursodeoxycholic acid** (a constituent of bile salts) dissolves the cholesterol gallstone and indirectly reduces cholesterol secretion into the bile by the liver. The net effect is a reduction in cholesterol concentration in the bile.

20. Nausea and emesis

Questions
- What are the major causes of nausea and vomiting?
- What drugs are used for the treatment of nausea and vomiting?

Nausea is a subjective unpleasant wave-like sensation experienced in the back of the throat and may or may not culminate in emesis, the forceful expulsion of contents of the gastrointestinal tract through the oral cavity. These physiological processes are a defensive mechanism to remove or avoid ingestion of harmful substances. Nausea and vomiting can occur as a result of gastrointestinal disturbances, pregnancy, motion sickness and intracranial pathology. They can also occur in postoperative nausea and vomiting (PONV), administration of drugs, cancer therapy (drug and radiation), antibiotics, analgesics (narcotics, NSAIDs) and following sensory stimuli (visual, auditory, olfactory, psychogenic). The control of emesis arises from the stimulation of two anatomically and functionally separate areas of the brainstem, the vomiting centre (VC) and a chemoreceptor trigger zone (CTZ) (Fig. 3.20.1). The CTZ responds to a variety of hormones, toxins and drugs within the circulation and to a rise in intracranial pressure. This region also receives afferent projections from mechanoreceptors and chemoreceptors from the gastrointestinal tract and other organs and peripheral pain receptors (Fig. 3.20.2). The VC is a collection of second-order neurons that receives input from the CTZ, vagal afferents and higher brain function (e.g. fear, anxiety). The VC is responsible for emesis involved in olfactory, emotional/anticipatory, hormonal/stress and pain-inducing vomiting.

Drug treatment
A number of drug classes are available that provide symptomatic relief against nausea and emesis. These can act centrally or peripherally at the gastrointestinal tract itself and include antagonists at $5HT_3$, dopamine (D_2), muscarinic and histamine receptors.

$5HT_3$ receptor antagonists
Ondansetron, **granisetron** and **tropisetron** block $5HT_3$ receptors both centrally (CTZ, NTS) and peripherally in the gastrointestinal tract and are, therefore, effective in emesis induced by emetogenic chemotherapeutic agents (e.g. cisplatin) and PONV. These stimuli lead to serotonin release within the gastrointestinal tract and centrally. These drugs are ineffective in motion sickness. They have few adverse reactions and their use can be accompanied by headache and constipation (blockade of $5HT_3$ receptors in the gastrointestinal tract).

Dopamine (D_2) receptor antagonists
A variety of dopamine agonists used in the treatment of Parkinson's disease, including apomorphine, levodopa, lergotrile and bromocriptine, induce nausea and emesis by an action on D_2 receptors in the CTZ and NTS. This effect is blocked by D_2 receptor antagonists, including **prochlorperazine**, **metoclopramide**, **domperidone**, **haloperidol** and **droperidol**. Extrapyramidal side-effects, including motor impairment, akinesia, muscle rigidity and dystonia (in children), can occur with the use of these agents. This can be minimized with domperidone, which has limited penetration into the CNS. This drug class is useful in emesis caused by opiates, PONV and emesis induced by chemotherapy or radiation, but higher doses are usually required.

Muscarinic receptor antagonists
Hyoscine butylbromide (**scopolamine**) is the most effective remedy for motion sickness, although nausea and emesis caused by severe vestibular disturbances (e.g. extreme changes in direction and space travel) are not treated. These drugs act on muscarinic receptors involved in afferent input from the

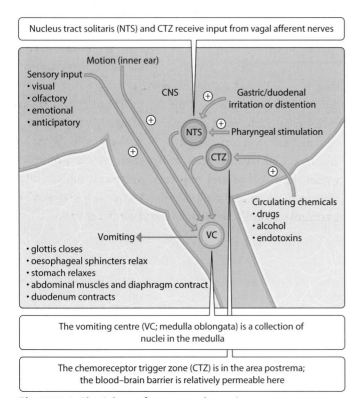

Nucleus tract solitaris (NTS) and CTZ receive input from vagal afferent nerves

Sensory input
- visual
- olfactory
- emotional
- anticipatory

Motion (inner ear)

CNS

Gastric/duodenal irritation or distention

NTS

Pharyngeal stimulation

CTZ

Circulating chemicals
- drugs
- alcohol
- endotoxins

Vomiting ◄   VC

- glottis closes
- oesophageal sphincters relax
- stomach relaxes
- abdominal muscles and diaphragm contract
- duodenum contracts

The vomiting centre (VC; medulla oblongata) is a collection of nuclei in the medulla

The chemoreceptor trigger zone (CTZ) is in the area postrema; the blood–brain barrier is relatively permeable here

Fig. 3.20.1 Physiology of nausea and emesis.

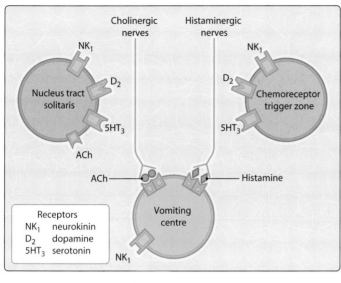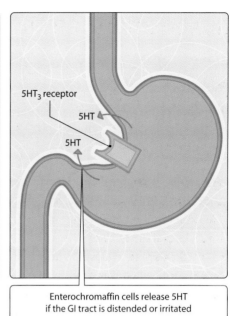

Fig. 3.20.2 Receptors involved in nausea and emesis.

gastrointestinal tract and the vestibular system to the VC. Adverse effects include sedation, dry mouth and blurred vision.

Antihistamines

Histamine H₁ receptor antagonists, including **promethazine**, **diphenhydramine**, **dimenhydrinate** and **cinnarizine**, act on the vestibular apparatus of the inner ear and are, therefore, useful in motion sickness and vomiting in vestibular disease. Most antihistamines have additional anticholinergic properties, which may also contribute toward the therapeutic action and side-effects (e.g. dry mouth) and sedation.

Phenothiazines

Phenothiazines including **chlorpromazine**, **promethazine**, **prochlorperazine** and **trimeprazine** are dopamine antagonists but also have muscarinic, histaminic, adrenergic and serotonergic antagonistic activity. These drugs act in the CTZ and VC and are, therefore, powerful anti-emetic agents. They are used to treat emesis and nausea caused by cytotoxic agents, radiation, opioids, migraine, pregnancy and PONV. Their mixed pharma-

cology also accounts for their side-effects, including dystonia in children, sedation and dry mouth.

Other agents

A synthetic derivative of **tetrahydrocannabinol** (active constituent of cannabis) is useful against nausea and emesis caused by cytotoxic chemotherapy that is unresponsive to other anti-emetics. Side-effects include drowsiness and dizziness. Corticosteroids including **dexamethasone** have been reported to have anti-emetic activity in patients undergoing chemotherapy. The general consensus is that combination of corticosteroids with other anti-emetic drug classes is more effective than single drug use. A new agent used for the treatment of nausea and vomiting associated with cancer chemotherapy is **aprepitant**, a neurokinin 1 receptor antagonist. Neurokinin 1 receptors are also found on vagal afferents in the gastrointestinal tract and within the NTS and area postrema. Aprepitant inhibits cytochrome P450 and should not be taken with terfenadine, astemizole, cisapride, warfarin and oral contraceptives.

21. Respiratory system: asthma

Questions
- What is asthma?
- What drugs are used for the treatment of asthma?

Asthma

Allergic asthma is the most common form of the disease (Fig. 3.21.1) but non-allergic asthma, which is not attributable to an allergic insult but results in a similar pathology and occurs later in life, is often more severe. Asthma can also develop following exposure to chemicals (e.g. isocyanates), when it is referred to as occupational asthma.

Drug treatment

Drug treatment usually involves providing symptomatic relief (bronchodilators) and preventative medication (glucocorticosteroids).

Bronchodilators

Beta 2 adrenoceptor agonists. Activation of β_2-adrenoceptors on airway smooth muscle results in elevated levels of intracellular cAMP, which activates protein kinase A and subsequently inhibits phosphorylation of myosin-like chain kinase, leading to relaxation. Activation of β_2-adrenoceptors on mast cells inhibits mast cell degranulation and the release of mediators (Fig. 3.21.1). These drugs (**salbutamol**, **terbutaline, fenoterol, formoterol** and **salmeterol**) provide rapid and effective relief against acute bronchoconstriction caused by a wide range of stimuli, including allergens (Fig. 3.21.2). Salbutamol, terbutaline and fenoterol have relatively short (4–6 h) while formoterol and salmeterol have longer (12–15 h) durations of action following a single inhaled dose. The longer-acting drugs are useful in preventing nocturnal awakenings owing to exacerbation of the underlying disease process in the early hours of the morning and are of great benefit in providing undisturbed sleep. Side-effects of this drug class include tremor, hypokalaemia and tachycardia, but these wane with regular usage.

Anticholinergic drugs. Muscarinic antagonists like **ipratropium bromide**, **oxitropium** and **tiotropium bromide** cause bronchodilatation by preventing the action of acetylcholine released from parasympathetic vagal nerves innervating the airways. They do not distinguish between different muscarinic subtypes and do not prevent all types of bronchospasm but are effective against bronchoconstriction induced by irritants (activating afferent nerves in the airways and causing reflex activation of parasympathetic nerves). They have modest action in asthma and are usually combined with β_2-adrenoceptor agonists. They are predominantly used in the treatment and management of chronic obstructive pulmonary disease.

Theophylline. Theophylline is a xanthine chemically related to caffeine, a constituent of coffee. Theophylline is administered orally but is a weak bronchodilator and has a narrow therapeutic window, which requires monitoring of plasma levels; side-effects including nausea, emesis, cardiac arrhythmias and convulsions. There are also important drug interactions that can increase (barbiturates, benzodiazepines) or decrease (cimetidine, erythromycin, ciprofloxacin) cytochrome P450 activity and metabolism of theophylline. Sustained-release preparations provide good

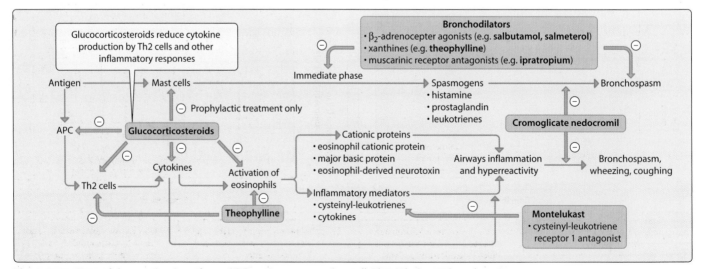

Fig. 3.21.1 Sites of drug action in asthma. APC, antigen-presenting cell; Th2, T helper 2 lymphocyte.

control of nocturnal asthma but should not be used to treat an acute exacerbation. Intravenous administration of aminophylline can be used to treat acute severe asthma. The mode of action of theophylline is not completely understood but may involve inhibition of phosphodiesterase, responsible for the hydrolysis of cAMP. This drug may have additional anti-inflammatory properties (see below).

Anti-inflammatory drugs

Glucocorticosteroids. **Beclometasone diproprionate, budesonide,** and **fluticasone propionate** are examples of inhaled glucocorticosteroids with anti-inflammatory properties (Fig. 3.21.2). The development of the late asthmatic response following inhalation of allergen is prevented by this drug class but they do not inhibit the early response. The molecular mechanism of action involves interfering with gene transcription of pro-inflammatory mediators and upregulating transcription of anti-inflammatory proteins (e.g. lipocortin). Their prolonged use diminishes airway hyperresponsiveness, mucus hypersecretion, oedema, local production of lipid-derived mediators, release of cytokines and reduced infiltration of eosinophils and mast cells. Glucocorticosteroids are administered by the inhaled route on a regular basis, although oral administration of prednisolone is advisable in chronic severe asthma. In status asthmaticus, intravenous administration of hydrocortisone is indicated. Common side-effects associated with inhaled glucocorticosteroids include thrush and dysphonia, which can be minimized by rinsing the mouth or by using spacer devices to increase drug deposition to the airway. Prolonged use of this drug class is associated with suppression of the hypothalamic–pituitary axis and loss in bone density, particularly when high doses are employed.

Anti-allergic drugs. **Sodium cromoglicate, nedocromil sodium** and **ketotifen** are examples of anti-allergic agents that have an anti-inflammatory activity, although glucocorticosteroids are superior in this regard (Fig. 3.21.2B). Their mechanism of action is not clear. They are weak mast cell-stabilizing agents but also have additional actions in suppressing the function of inflammatory cells. They are not used to treat acute symptoms and must be taken on a regular basis. Ketotifen has additional antihistamine properties and is useful in young patients. Ketotifen, is orally bioavailable.

Theophylline. Theophylline has bronchodilatory activity but when administered over prolonged periods demonstrates anti-inflammatory activity. Inhibition of phosphodiesterase activity in inflammatory cells may be involved.

Cysteinyl-leukotriene antagonists. **Montelukast** is a once a day orally available drug that inhibits the actions of cysteinyl-leukotrienes on effector cells, including airway smooth muscle. It has some usefulness in the treatment of aspirin-sensitive asthma and asthma exacerbated by exercise, and to reduce the incidence of nocturnal awakenings.

Omlizumab. A monoclonal antibody against human IgE has been shown to reduce airway inflammation and symptoms in severe asthma. This biological treatment is expensive and needs to be administered systemically.

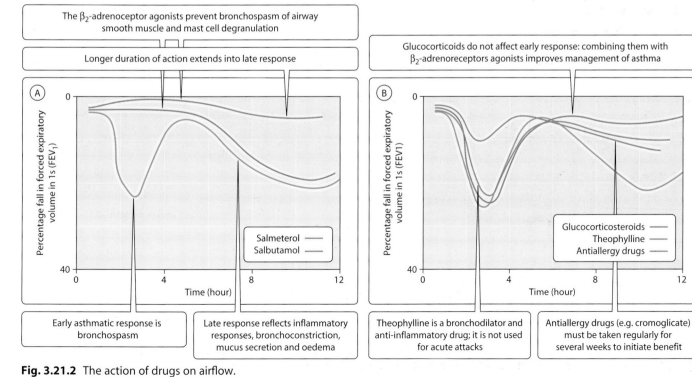

Fig. 3.21.2 The action of drugs on airflow.

22. Respiratory system: chronic obstructive pulmonary disease

Questions
- What is chronic obstructive pulmonary disease?
- What drugs are used for its treatment?

Chronic obstructive pulmonary disease (COPD) is characterized by airflow obstruction that is partly reversible and progressively deteriorates. Those who suffer from COPD have reduced lung function (as expressed by forced expiratory volume in one second; FEV_1) and exacerbation of symptoms (including cough and mucus secretion). Because of the nature of this disease, subjects can suffer from a diminished capacity to undertake physical exertion and have a poor quality of life.

Cigarette smoking and exposure to indoor pollution (e.g. smoke from burning of biomass fuels) are major factors in its morbidity (Fig. 3.22.1). Smoking cessation should be encouraged because it is the only form of 'treatment' that has been shown to reduce disease progression. However, this can be difficult for a majority of smokers because of nicotine addiction. It is, therefore, of interest that the antidepressant **bupropion** given for a short period improves the likelihood of smoking abstinence.

Drug treatment
A number of pharmacological agents are used in the management of COPD but none halts the accelerated decline in the lung function seen in this disease.

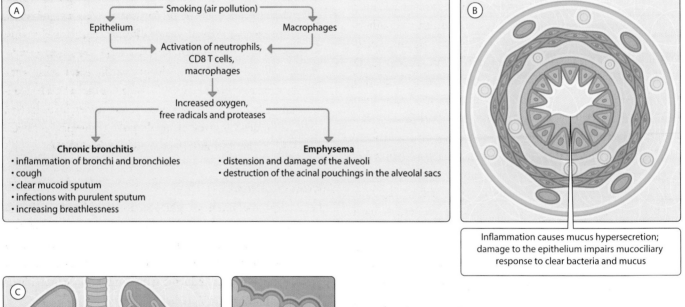

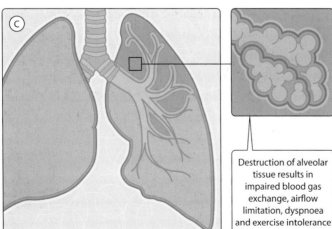

Fig. 3.22.1 Chronic obstructive pulmonary disease. (A) Pathophysiology; (B) a bronchiole in bronchitis; (C) emphysema.

Bronchodilators

Bronchodilator drugs can improve airflow obstruction but the poorly reversible nature of the obstruction in this disease means that only variable increases in baseline FEV_1 will be demonstrated. However, the benefit to the patient comes in the form of an increase in ventilation at a lower functional residual capacity and reducing hyperinflation, which improves the capacity to exercise.

Anticholinergic drugs. Anticholinergic drugs including **ipratropium bromide**, **oxitropium bromide** and **tiotropium bromide** antagonize the actions of acetylcholine release from parasympathetic nerves innervating the lung. As a consequence airway smooth muscle relaxation and inhibition of mucus secretion are desirable beneficial actions. Muscarinic M_2 receptors are found on the terminal ending of parasympathetic nerves and activation of these receptors leads to a reduction in the release of acetylcholine from parasympathetic nerves. In contrast, activation of M_3 receptors on effector cells like airway smooth muscle leads to contraction. It would be desirable to antagonize the actions of acetylcholine selectively at M_3 but not M_2 receptors, as the latter act as a negative feedback mechanism to limit the release of acetylcholine from parasympathetic terminals. Ipratropium bromide is a non-selective antagonist but nonetheless is effective in the treatment of COPD. However, its short duration of action necessitates self-medication on a regular basis. In contrast, tiotropium bromide has affinity for both receptor subtypes but appears to dissociate rapidly from M_2 receptors while remaining firmly bound to the M_3 receptor and, as a consequence, has a prolonged duration of action (once daily treatment). Tiotropium bromide significantly improves lung function, reduces symptoms, increases quality of life and reduces exacerbation rates.

Beta-2 adrenoceptor agonists. Relaxation of airway smooth muscle can also be induced by β_2-adrenoceptor agonists (e.g. **salbutamol**, **salmeterol** and **formoterol**). Coupling of β_2-adrenoceptors with G-protein activates the effector protein adenylyl cyclase in airway smooth muscle leading to a rise in intracellular levels of cAMP; this, in turn, activates protein kinase A and ultimately causes relaxation of the airway smooth muscle. Both salmeterol and formoterol are superior to salbutamol in terms of duration of action and as such improve lung function, reduce symptoms and increase the quality of life in COPD. Though shorter-acting, salbutamol offers the advantage of providing rapid bronchodilator relief and, therefore, is commonly prescribed as rescue medication during an exacerbation of disease. Unlike the anticholinergic drugs, β_2-adrenoceptor agonists do not inhibit mucus secretion; however, they have been shown to improve mucociliary clearance and inhibit neutrophil function, although to what extent these other actions contribute to the clinical efficacy of this drug class is not clear at present. The difference in bronchodilator mechanism between anticholinergic and β_2-adrenoceptor agonists suggests that combination therapy is appropriate for the management of COPD and may also apply to combination therapy with long-acting β_2-adrenoceptor agonists and tiotropium bromide.

Theophylline. Its usefulness in COPD is limited because of the greater side-effects associated with this drug. Theophylline can relax airway smooth muscle, albeit at high concentrations. It has been proposed that theophylline elevates cAMP within cells following inhibition of phosphodiesterase. However, this drug is a weak phosphodiesterase inhibitor and it is not surprising that the doses required for bronchodilatation result in side-effects of nausea and emesis. Interestingly, theophylline also has anti-neutrophilic activity and, therefore, could potentially exert some anti-inflammatory action in COPD. Whether the action of theophylline can be improved is currently under investigation with the development of highly potent phosphodiesterase (PDE) 4 inhibitors as potential therapy for COPD.

Glucocorticosteroids

The clinical usefulness of glucocorticosteroids in COPD is controversial because long-term studies have shown that this drug class does not reduce the decline in lung function that is characteristic of this disease. However, glucocorticosteroids may provide some benefit in reducing symptoms in those individuals who have an $FEV_1 < 50\%$ predicted.

Supplementation with oxygen

There is no effective treatment for emphysema and individuals with severe reduction in FEV_1 usually require supplementation with oxygen.

23. Respiratory system: rhinitis

Questions
- What is allergic rhinitis?
- What drugs are used for the treatment of rhinitis?

Rhinitis is a common and debilitating disease characterized by rhinorrhoea, sneezing, itching nasal congestion and obstruction. Allergic rhinitis is a common form of this disease, and symptoms arise following acute exposure to allergen, which binds to cell surface-bound IgE on mast cells and triggers their degranulation and release of inflammatory mediators such as histamine, tryptase, cysteinyl-leukotrienes and cytokines. This acute response triggers symptoms of itching, sneezing, rhinorrhoea and nasal congestion (Fig. 3.23.1). A delayed recruitment of lymphocytes and eosinophils to the nasal mucosa, and the mediators released from these cells, is also thought to contribute towards these symptoms, although nasal congestion and obstruction predominate. Non-allergic rhinitis is not caused by an airborne allergen and symptoms might be triggered by viral infection, hormonal imbalance or vasomotor, occupational or drug causes. Allergy avoidance can minimize the symptoms of allergic rhinitis but this has many disadvantages as it requires a change in lifestyle, which is impracticable for many. There are a number of pharmacological approaches for the treatment of allergic rhinitis (Fig. 3.23.1B).

Pharmacological treatments

Antihistamines
Antihistamines are the most frequently used drugs in the treatment of allergic rhinitis. Histamine released from mast cells acts on a number of cells within the nasal mucosa resulting in symptoms of itching, sneezing (sensory nerves), rhinorrhoea and mucus secretion (submucosal glands). These drugs are less effective in reducing nasal congestion. First-generation anti-

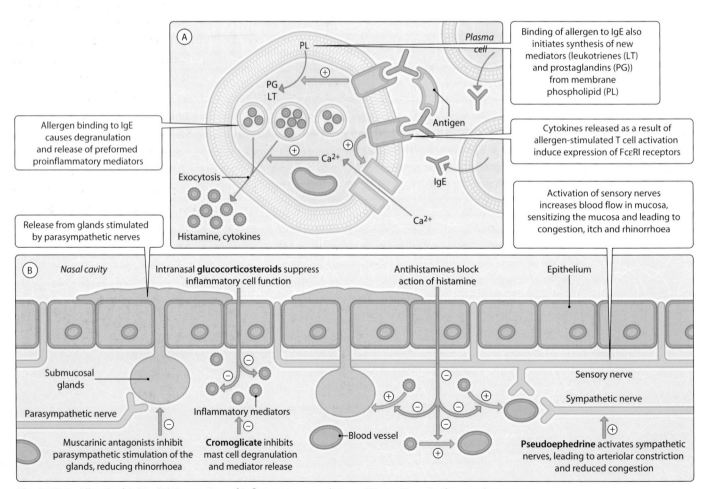

Fig. 3.23.1 Allergic rhinitis. (A) Formation of inflammatory mediators; (B) reactions in the nasal passages.

histamines such as **diphenhydramine** and **chlorpheniramine** cross the blood–brain barrier and cause drowsiness; the incidence of this side-effect was reduced with second-generation antihistamines **terfenadine** and **astemizole**; however, these drugs produced potentially fatal cardiac arrhythmias in some patients. Newer antihistamines such as **loratidine** and **fexofenadine** are non-sedating, non-cardiotoxic and have long duration of action. As such, these drugs are administered orally. Intranasal preparations are available and include **azelastine**, which provides rapid relief. Some antihistamines also have a mild anti-inflammatory action (e.g. **cetirizine**).

Sympathomimetic drugs

Oral decongestants include **pseudoephedrine** (indirect acting) and **phenylephrine** (direct acting) and may also be used to decrease the swelling of the nasal mucosa by stimulating vasoconstriction. However, this class is only used for short periods (not more than 3 days) because of the potential for rebound increase in nasal congestion when discontinued.

Anticholinergic drugs

Parasympathetic stimulation of the nasal glands gives rise to a watery secretion and symptoms of rhinorrhoea. Topical administration of **ipratropium bromide** to the nose is effective in reducing the watery discharge, particularly prominent in perennial rhinitis. These drugs do not affect nasal congestion, sneezing or itch.

Anti-allergic drugs

Mast cell degranulation following antigen cross-linking with surface bound IgE is inhibited by **disodium cromoglicate** and **nedocromil sodium**. These drugs are effective when applied topically to the nasal surface. **Ketotifen** has a similar profile of activity and is administered orally. These agents are not used to suppress acute symptoms and generally are prophylactic, preferably initiated prior to the commencement of the pollen season. They may also have additional anti-inflammatory properties and are more effective in children.

Glucocorticosteroids

Glucocorticosteroids are the mainstay of therapy for allergic and non-allergic rhinitis. They reduce vascular permeability, the recruitment and activity of inflammatory cells and the secretion of cytokines and synthesis of lipid-derived mediators. These drugs can be administered topically (e.g. **flunisolide**, **beclometasone dipropionate**, **triamcinolone acetonide** and **fluticasone propionate**). They reduce all the symptoms of rhinitis, including congestion, sneezing, rhinorrhoea and itching, with improvement in symptoms occurring after prophylactic treatment (i.e. after several weeks). In severe rhinitis, glucocorticosteroids may also be given systemically. In these circumstances, prednisolone is useful. Combination with antihistamines may be employed in moderate-to-severe rhinitis.

Other therapies

Immunotherapy involves giving gradually increasing doses of the substance (or allergen) to which the person is allergic. This makes the immune system less sensitive to that substance, probably by causing production of a particular 'blocking' antibody, which reduces the symptoms of allergy when the substance is encountered in the future. Before starting treatment, the physician and patient try to identify trigger factors for allergic symptoms. Skin or sometimes blood tests are performed to confirm the specific allergens to which the person has antibodies. This treatment is indicated when allergen avoidance or pharmacotherapy has failed to suppress symptoms adequately. The treatment is expensive, requires identification of the offending insult and frequent visits and there is a potential for anaphylactic reactions. One emerging therapeutic agent is **omalizumab**, a monoclonal IgE antibody that binds to circulating IgE. Administered s.c., it has been shown to reduce nasal symptoms significantly and improve quality of life during the pollen season; this is associated with a fall in circulating levels of IgE. The cysteinyl-leukotriene antagonist **montelukast** has been approved for use in the USA for the treatment of allergic rhinitis and improves daytime and night-time symptoms and reduces the action of cysteinyl-leukotrienes on the nasal mucosa.

24. Thyroid disorders

Questions
- What are some examples of thyroid disorders?
- What are the treatments for these disorders?

The thyroid hormones triiodothyronine (T_3) and thyroxine (T_4) play an important role in development (physical and cognitive), metabolism (carbohydrate, lipid, protein), body temperature regulation and have a direct action on various organs (e.g. increased cardiac function) (Fig. 3.24.1). In hyperthyroidism (or thyrotoxicosis), there is an endogenous overproduction or excessive ingestion of thyroid hormones. Examples include Graves' disease (diffuse toxic goitre), thyroiditis, thyroid-stimulating hormone (TSH)-secreting adenoma, and multinodular goitre. Graves' disease is an autoimmune disease caused by TSH antibodies, which bind to and activate TSH receptors on target cells. A characteristic feature of Graves' disease is protruding eyes caused by binding of the TSH antibody to a TSH receptor-like protein in the retro-orbital connective tissue, leading to swelling in muscle and connective tissue behind the eye. Other symptoms of hyperthyroidism are a result of the increase in metabolic rate, resulting in increased skin temperature, sweating, weight loss, tremor and palpitation, owing in part to excessive β-adrenoceptor stimulation. In contrast, hypothyroidism is a failure by the thyroid to synthesize and release thyroid hormones. Examples include Hashimoto's thyroiditis, atrophic thyroiditis, postablative therapy, iodine deficiency and genetic disorders involving the synthesis of thyroid hormone. Hashimoto's thyroiditis is an autoimmune disease caused by production of antithyroid antibodies (e.g. antithyroid peroxidase, antithyroglobulin). Symptoms include lethargy, cold intolerance, weight gain and constipation. A lifelong impairment in cognition and abnormal skeletal muscle development is a characteristic feature of cretinism.

Antithyroid drugs

Thioureylenes. A number of drugs including **carbimazole**, **methimazole** and **propylthiouracil** are first-line drugs for the treatment of hyperthyroidism. These thiourea compounds are actively transported into the thyroid and inhibit thyroid peroxidase activity, thereby leading to a reduction in synthesis and storage of thyroid hormones. Carbimazole is converted to methimazole and both drugs are administered once daily and have a faster onset of action than propylthiouracil, although they may take several weeks to deplete stored thyroid hormone. Propylthiouracil has the additional property of blocking the peripheral conversion of T_4 to T_3 thereby inhibiting the peripheral action of thyroid hormone. Side-effects of this drug class are pruritus, rash, fever, nausea and agranulocytosis, although the last is rare. An acute exacerbation of thyrotoxicosis is referred to as a thyroid storm and can be treated with thionamides, iodine and beta-blockers (see later).

Anion transport inhibitors. A variety of anions competitively interfere with the accumulation of iodine into the thyroid cell, thereby blocking the synthesis of thyroxine. Iodide (supersaturated potassium iodide solution, Lugol's solution) is a rapid treatment for hyperthyroidism (1–2 days) as it inhibits the synthesis of T_3 and T_4. However, this effect is transient, lasting only a couple of weeks. Another effect of high plasma concentrations of circulating iodine is suppression of thyroid hormone release from this cell. This form of treatment is used preoperatively in preparing affected individuals who are scheduled for thyroidectomy and in the management of thyroid storm.

Radioactive iodine. The administration of I^{131} (oral in solution or as a capsule) is an effective cure for hyperthyroidism, with permanent hypothyroidism being inevitable in virtually all patients. The selective transport of the β-emitting radionucleotide into the thyroid produces thyroiditis. It is useful in patients with Graves' disease or those with toxic nodules or toxic multinodular goitre. Cessation of treatment with antithyroid drugs should occur prior to treatment to avoid preventing uptake of the iodine into the thyroid. This form of treatment is contraindicated in pregnancy.

Thyroidectomy. Surgery is only used in certain circumstances for the treatment of hyperthyroidism, including patient preference, poor response to antithyroid drugs and presence of a large goitre or malignant thyroid nodule. Before surgery, patients are given iodine in order to inhibit thyroid hormone production and release and to reduce blood flow to the gland, which will facilitate surgical removal of the organ. Hypothyroidism is a natural consequence of this procedure.

Beta-blockers. These agents do not suppress thyroid hormone production, although some beta-blockers do appear to inhibit the conversion of T_4 to T_3 in peripheral tissues. They are used to suppress the increased β-adrenergic activity (palpitations, tachycardia, tremor and heat intolerance) associated with hyperthyroidism.

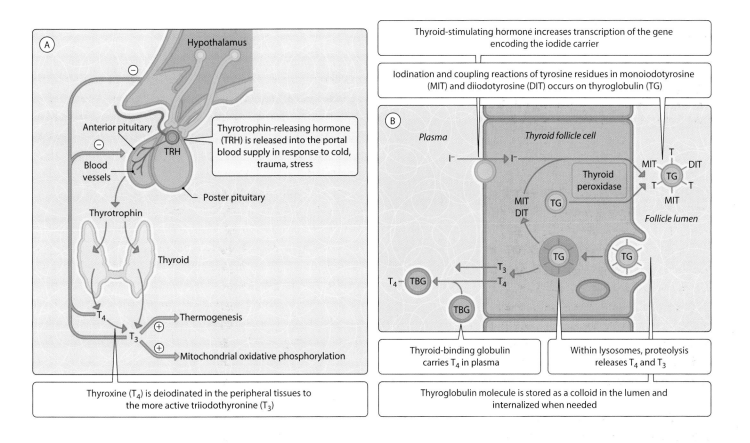

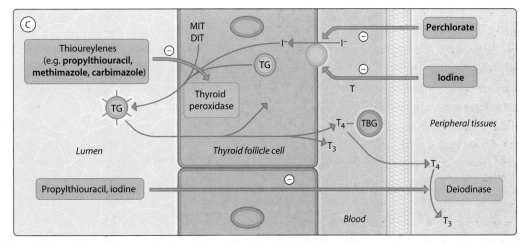

Fig. 3.24.1 Regulation of thyroid hormone production. (A) Feedback control; (B) thyroid hormone synthesis; (C) modulation by drugs.

Treatment of hypothyroidism

Replacement thyroxine (synthetic **levothyroxine**) or **liothyronine** (sodium salt of T_3) is the mainstay treatment for hypothyroidism. The half-life of thyroxine is 1 week and, therefore, once daily administration is sufficient to maintain adequate plasma levels. Normalization of plasma TSH levels is the best biochemical marker of treatment in primary hypothyroidism. In hypothalamopituitary hypothyroidism (secondary hypothyroidism), serum TSH is not a valid biochemical marker of treatment and serum levels of T_4 must be monitored.

25. Diabetes mellitus

Questions
- What is diabetes mellitus?
- What are the treatments for this disorder?

The stimulation of glucose uptake in peripheral tissue (e.g. skeletal muscle and adipose tissue) is an important function of insulin (see Fig. 1.12). The inability to regulate plasma glucose in the normal physiological range is central to diabetes mellitus, accounting for the hyperglycaemia, increase in thirst (polydipsia), increased glucose in urine (glycosuria) and large volumes of dilute urine (polyuria). High plasma glucose leads to retinal disease, peripheral nerve dysfunction, atherosclerosis and peripheral vascular disease. Type I diabetes is an autoimmune disease that leads to the destruction of pancreatic beta cells in the young. In contrast, type II diabetes affects adults and has a number of predisposing factors, including genetics, obesity and sedentary lifestyle. It is also characterized by impaired insulin secretion from pancreatic beta cells coupled with an inability of peripheral cells to respond to insulin, commonly referred to as insulin resistance. The mechanism of this resistance include defects in glucose transport mechanism, glucotoxicity and lipotoxicity. The release of insulin from beta cells of the pancreas is regulated by plasma glucose (Figs 3.25.1 and 3.25.2) and a range of pharmacological agents can be used to reduce hyperglycaemia in diabetes mellitus (Fig. 3.25.3).

Insulin

Insulin is used to treat type I diabetes, reducing hepatic glucose production and improving glucose utilization by skeletal muscle. The biological activity of insulin is impaired by the gastrointestinal tract and it must, therefore, be given s.c., although in emergency it is administered i.v. There are many insulin formulations that slow absorption from the injection site, resulting in different times to reach peak insulin levels and duration of action (e.g. short-acting (e.g. regular, semilente), intermediate (e.g. lente, neutral protamine (isophane) insulin) and long-acting

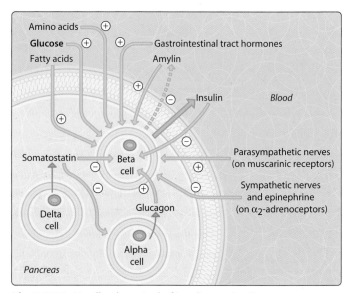

Fig. 3.25.1 Feedback control of insulin production.

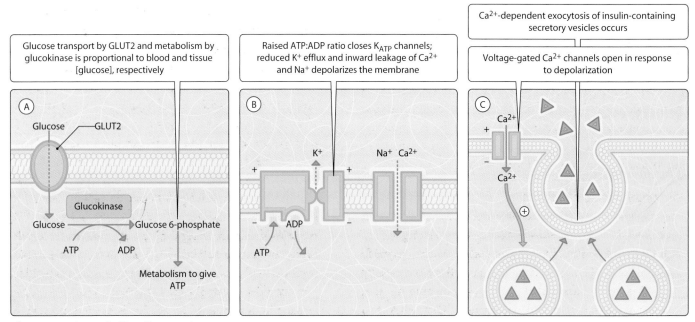

Fig. 3.25.2 Control of insulin secretion.

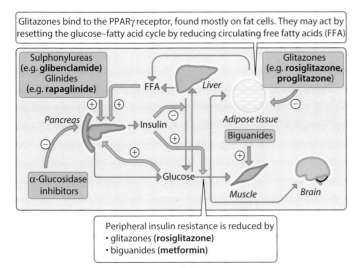

Glitazones bind to the PPARγ receptor, found mostly on fat cells. They may act by resetting the glucose–fatty acid cycle by reducing circulating free fatty acids (FFA)

Fig. 3.25.3 Drugs used to treat diabetes.

(ultralente) insulin). These allow the patient some flexibility in matching calorific intake with lifestyles. Regular insulin consists of crystalline zinc insulin that is injected 30 min before a meal, resulting in peak plasma levels of insulin within 2 to 3 h and an effect that lasts for 6 h. Insulin lispro and Insulin aspart are genetically engineered recombinant monomeric forms that do not dimerize and, therefore, are more rapidly absorbed; they are administered just prior to a meal. Because of their short duration of action, these monomeric analogues produce less hypoglycaemia than regular insulin. Intermediate preparations consist of large insulin crystals prepared in buffer or with addition of protamine in order to reduce solubility. Morphous zinc insulin and insulin zinc crystals in acetate buffer (lente) or insulin in a phosphate buffer together with protamine (NPH) allow insulin to dissolve more slowly from the site of injection, giving a more gradual onset (peak 6–10 h) and prolonged duration (20 h). Similarly, ultralente insulin consists of poorly soluble insulin zinc crystals that results in peak plasma levels within 20 h and a duration of 30 h. An important unwanted effect of insulin is hypoglycaemia, which can result in insufficient plasma glucose to meet the demands of the central nervous system, pontentially causing brain damage. Hypoglycaemia can be avoided by eating a sweet snack or drink or an infusion of glucose can be administered if the patient is unconscious.

Oral hypoglycaemic drugs

Sulphonylureas. Insulin secretion by the pancreatic beta cell is controlled by ATP-sensitive potassium channels (Fig. 3.25.2). **Tolbutamide** (first generation) and **gibenclamide**, **glipizide** and **glicazide** (second generation) block these channels by binding to an associated sulphonylurea-binding site, resulting in membrane depolarization, Ca^{2+} entry and insulin secretion. These drugs not only stimulate insulin secretion in fasting states but also augment insulin secretion

after ingestion of a meal. Sulphonylureas are not effective in patients with severe beta cell dysfunction or in pancreatized diabetes. Potential disadvantages include hypoglycaemia, the incidence of which is dependent on the potency and duration of action of the drug. Weight gain is another unwanted action as this drug class stimulates appetite, which can be a potential issue in obese patients.

Non-sulphonylurea secretagogues. These stimulate secretion of insulin from pancreatic beta cells by inhibiting the ATP-sensitive potassium channel but act at sites distinct from the sulphonylurea-binding site. The glinides (**repaglinide**, **nateglinide**) have shorter half-lives than sulphonylureas and provide a brief stimulation of insulin secretion; they are most effective during the post-prandial state. Potential disadvantages include hypoglycaemia, weight gain and the requirement for frequent dosing.

Biguanides. The biguanide **metformin** inhibits hepatic glucose production and improves insulin resistance by a poorly understood mechanism, but nonetheless it alleviates hyperglycaemia in type II diabetes. Biguanides do not stimulate insulin secretion and, therefore, do not produce hypoglycaemia, weight gain or exacerbate hyperinsulinaemia. Because of these advantages, metformin is usually the drug of first choice. It is also used in combination with sulphonylureas. There is a risk of metabolic acidosis, abdominal bloating and diarrhoea, and biguanides are contraindicated in patients with renal insufficiency, hepatic dysfunction and congestive heart failure.

Thiazolidinediones (glitazones). These drugs (e.g. **rosiglitazone** and **pioglitazone**) are ligands for the peroxisome proliferator activator receptors (PPARγ), activation of which alters gene transcription, particularly those involved in carbohydrate and lipid metabolism (e.g. lipoprotein lipase, GLUT4). PPARγ are found in skeletal muscle and liver but particularly in adipocytes. Their stimulation reduces plasma glucose and fatty acid levels via promotion of glucose uptake in muscle, reduction of hepatic glucose production and increased fatty acid uptake/storage in adipocytes. All increases the effectiveness of endogenous insulin (reduces insulin resistance). These drugs do not induce hypoglycaemia but cause weight gain and fluid retention the latter of concern in patients with congestive heart failure.

Alpha-glucosidase inhibitors. Inhibitors like **acarbose** and **miglitol** specifically target α-glucosidase within the brush border of gastrointestinal tract epithelium. This enzyme breaks down complex carbohydrates so its competitive inhibition delays carbohydrate absorption and reduces the increase in postprandial glucose levels but fasting glucose levels are little affected. Side-effects include flatulence, abdominal discomfort and diarrhoea.

26. Adrenal corticosteroids

Questions
- What is the physiological role of adrenal corticosteroids?
- When are endogenous and synthetic corticosteroids used?

Corticosteroids are synthesized in the adrenal cortex under the control of the hypothalamic–pituitary axis (Fig. 3.26.1); and play an important role in carbohydrate and protein metabolism (glucocorticosteroids) and electrolyte balance (mineralcorticosteroids). The endogenous corticosteroid hydrocortisone (cortisol) demonstrates potency for both these activities and greater selectivity for glucocorticosteroid activity has been achieved with a variety of synthetic analogues, which are utilized clinically to treat inflammatory conditions. Aldosterone (mineralcorticosteroid) is secreted from the adrenal cortex following activation of the renin–angiotensin system and promotes Na^+ reabsorption, water retention and K^+ excretion (see Fig. 3.17.1). Corticosteroids bind to intracellular receptors that translocate to the nucleus of cells and bind to corticosteroid response elements (CRE) upstream of promoter region of genes, thereby influencing their rate of transcription.

Glucocorticosteroids

Glucocorticosteroids mainly affect the metabolism of carbohydrates (promote gluconeogenesis in the liver), lipids (enhance lipolysis by lipolytic agents) and protein (increase protein breakdown).

Impaired production

Deficiencies in the synthesis of hydrocortisone (e.g. Addison's disease) give rise to a number of life-threatening symptoms including weakness, lethargy, susceptibility to infection (lack of glucocorticosteroid activity), hypotension, dehydration and excessive loss of Na^+ (lack of mineralcorticosteroid activity). Impairment of the hypothalamic–pituitary axis also gives rise to these symptoms. In defective adrenocorticothalamic hormone (ACTH) secretion, the body can still synthesize aldosterone as this is under the control of the renin–angiotensin system. Deficiency disorders are treated with replacement therapy consisting of **hydrocortisone** (cortisol) or a synthetic glucocorticosteroid together with a mineralcorticosteroid twice daily in order to mimic the physiological rhythm of hormone release.

Excessive production

Cushing's syndrome is caused by excessive release of glucocorticosteroid

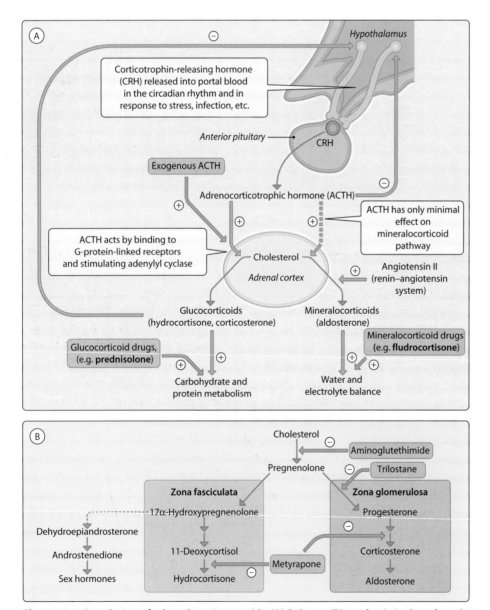

Fig. 3.26.1 Regulation of adrenal corticosteroids. (A) Release; (B) synthesis in the adrenal glands.

(e.g. from an ACTH-secreting adenoma in the pituitary gland). The characteristic features are easily explained from the physiological action of the glucocorticosteroids: central obesity with the appearance of a moon-shaped face (redistribution of fat); hyperglycaemia, which can lead to diabetes mellitus; osteoporosis (catabolism of protein matrix in bone); growth retardation in children and reduced linear bone growth (suppression of the hypothalamic–pituitary axis); loss of supporting structure in the skin resulting in atrophy, bruising and poor wound healing; muscle wasting and weakness; peptic ulceration (decreased prostaglandin synthesis); changes in mood; increased susceptibility to infection by bacteria, fungi and virus; and activation of latent infection (e.g. tuberculosis). Cushing's disease is treated by surgical removal of the adenoma from the pituitary. If the production of ACTH by a carcinoma is not amenable to surgery, control of excessive corticosteroid secretion can be achieved with **aminoglutethimide**, which inhibits 20α-hydroxylation of cholesterol, a rate-limiting step in the biosynthesis of steroids, and aromatase, which converts androgens to oestrogens. Mitotane has a selective cytotoxic action on adrenocortical cells and is reserved for the treatment of adrenal tumours. Inhibitors of steroid synthesis cause adverse drug reactions as the enzymes affected belong to the P450 family.

Non-endocrine effects

Glucocorticosteroids are also used in inflammatory conditions (Table 3.26.1). The development of more potent glucocorticosteroids has increased the potential for unwanted side-effects owing to systemic absorption, because of the ubiquity of glucocorticosteroid receptors throughout the body. However, this can be substantially diminished by delivering pharmacological relevant doses of glucocorticosteroid directly to the inflammatory site in the form of suppositories, creams or aerosol. Cortisol may be administered orally or i.v. for anaphylactic shock or status asthmaticus.

Mineralcorticosteroids

Aldosterone is secreted from the adrenal cortex and the principal target is the distal tubule of the kidney, where it increases the absorption of Na^+ by increasing the expression and function of Na^+ transporters and pumps. Aldosterone binds to steroid receptors and as a complex with the receptor

Table 3.26.1 CORTICOSTEROID THERAPY

Corticosteroid	GC activity	MC activity	Indication
Hydrocortisone Oral Intravenous Suppository	+	+	Corticosteroid replacement therapy Status asthmaticus, anaphylaxis Ulcerative colitis
Prednisolone Oral Intravenous Suppository Aqueous solution	+	–	Allergy and inflammatory conditions As oral use Ulcerative colitis Superficial ocular inflammation
Dexamethasone Oral Intravenous Aqueous solution	+	–	Allergic conditions Reduce cerebral oedema Superficial ocular inflammation
Beclomethasone, budesonide, fluticasone propionate (topical)	+++	–	Asthma, rhinitis (aerosol), eczma (cream)
Fludrocortisone (oral)	–	++	Addison's disease

GC, glucocorticoid; MC, mineralcorticoid.

translocates to the nucleus to increase expression of the genes for aldosterone-inducible proteins (AIP), which include Na^+/K^+-ATPase and Na^+ channels.

Aldosterone suffers from extensive first pass metabolism and is, therefore, unsuitable for oral use. **Fludrocortisone** is a synthetic alternative that is administered as replacement therapy in patients with defective aldosterone production. It is used in Addison's disease (autoimmune disease of adrenal cortex) together with a glucocorticosteroid (the latter to treat the symptoms of glucocorticosteroid deficiency).

In primary hyperaldosteronism (Conn's syndrome), excessive aldosterone secretion from an adenoma in the adrenal cortex results in salt and fluid retention, hypertension and hypokalaemia. Treatment is surgical removal and administration of K^+-sparing diuretics (e.g. **spironolactone**, **amiloride**).

27. Sex hormones: female

Questions
- How is female gonadal hormone secretion regulated?
- What are the major uses of female sex hormones?

The sex hormones oestrogen (17β-oestradiol, oestrone) and progesterone have important physiological actions in female development, regulation of ovulation and preparation of the female reproductive organ for fertilization and implantation. The secretion of gonadotrophin-releasing hormone (GnRH) from the hypothalamus is pulsatile in nature and under the control of a neural oscillator (or 'clock') (Fig. 3.27.1A). This hormone activates cells within the anterior pituitary to release luteinizing hormone (LH) and follicle-stimulating hormone (FSH), which regulate the growth and development of the Graafian follicle in the ovary, stimulate the release of oestrogen from the ovary to induce the proliferation of the endometrium in preparation for implantation, and provide feedback control on the release of gonadotrophins from the anterior pituitary (thus preventing the development of other less mature follicles). As the concentration of oestrogen rises, it exerts a positive feedback on the hypothalamus and pituitary, which promotes a surge in FSH and LH release, thus promoting ovulation (Fig. 3.26.1B). The ruptured follicle develops into the corpus luteum and secretes progesterone, which has negative feedback effects upon FSH release from the anterior pituitary by decreasing the GnRH pulse frequency, which also decreases LH pulse frequency, but

the *amplitude* of the pulses of LH is initially high (i.e. large amount released). Progesterone serves to diminish the proliferative effects of oestrogen upon the endometrium and stimulates differentiation of these cells. Mucus secretion and increased vascularization prepare the uterus for implantation. In the absence of fertilization, the corpus luteum regresses, oestrogen and progesterone levels fall and the endometrium cannot be maintained, resulting in menstruation. The biological activities of these sex hormones are mediated by binding to the steroid receptor family (oestrogen receptor and progestogen receptor).

Oral contraception
Oral contraceptives prevent the development of the Graafian follicle essentially by mimicking the physiological response that occurs during the luteal phase. The administration of oestradiol (**ethinylestrogen**) and progesterone (combined pill) inhibit gonadotrophin release from the anterior pituitary thus preventing the LH surge and consequently ovulation. Biphasic or triphasic preparations are used to reduce the overall dose of oestrogen/progestogens and to match more closely the endogenous levels of these hormones:

- monophasic: ethinylestradiol with one of the following, **norethindrone, levonorgestrel, norethindrone, desogestrel, norgestimate**
- biphasic: **ethinylestradiol** with **norethindrone**
- triphasic: **ethinylestradiol** with one of the following, **norethindrone, norgestimate** or **levonorgestrel**.

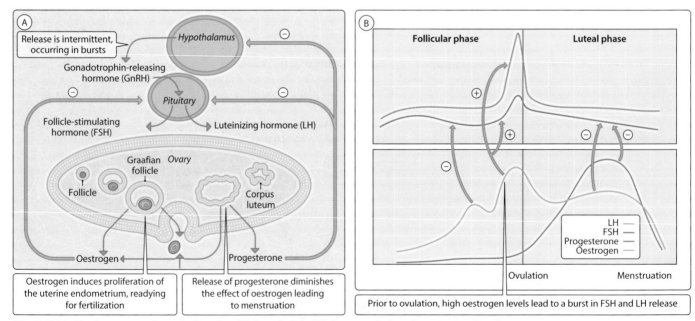

Fig. 3.27.1 Sex hormone release in females. (A) Regulation; (B) changes during the menstrual cycle.

Oestrogen suffers from extensive first pass metabolism, which is prevented by the ethinyl substitution. Administration by transdermal patches provides a slower and more sustained release. **Estradiol valerate** or **estradiol cypionate** (i.m.) provides an alternative slow-release method. In emergency, high-dose oestrogen can be used as postcoital pill to prevent egg implantation.

The advantages of oral contraceptives include reduced incidence of premenstrual tension, suppression of benign breast cancer, suppression of ovarian cysts and reduced risk of ovarian cancer; the disadvantages are thrombosis (only seen with high doses of oestrogens) and a suggested increased risk in breast cancer in some women (not proven). Weight gain, breakthrough bleeding and changes in mood/libido can occur.

Hormone replacement therapy

The consequences of the menopause include osteoporosis with increased incidence of bone fracture, vasomotor instability (e.g. hot flushes, night sweats), vaginitis (inflammation) and cardiovascular changes (increase in LDL cholesterol). Oestrogen replacement therapy relieves and reduces the risk of these symptoms. It is common to use naturally derived oestrogen (e.g. plant derived) conjugated with formulations of oestradiol. It is usual to administer with a progestogen (e.g. **medroxyprogesterone acetate**) as this counters the potential for the development of neoplasms in the endometrium. A number of adverse events associated with hormone replacement therapy include deep vein thrombosis, fluid retention, breast tenderness and a slight increased risk of breast cancer.

Anti-oestrogens

Anti-oestrogens (e.g. **tamoxifen**) are useful for the treatment of breast cancer and female infertility (Fig. 3.27.2). Oestrogen is a well-known risk factor for breast and uterine tumours. Anti-oestrogens inhibit the growth of these tumour cells, behaving as oestrogen receptor antagonists in the breast and pituitary and as partial agonists in other tissues (e.g. bone, endometrium).

Raloxifene is known as a 'selective oestrogen receptor modulator' (SERM) and behaves as an oestogen agonist in bone (increasing osteoblast activity); it is, therefore, used in the treatment of osteoporosis. Its actions as an oestrogen antagonist reduce the risk of breast cancer. **Clomiphene** inhibits oestrogen binding to its receptor in the pituitary, thereby preventing negative feedback inhibition of GnRH by endogenous oestrogen. This property is exploited in infertile women to increase the release of GnRH and encourage development of the ovaries in ovulation. Alternatively, the pulsatile injection of synthetic GnRH agonists (e.g. **nafarelin, goserelin**) can mimic the endogenous actions of GnRH and this approach is used to treat infertility caused by a failure of the pituitary to secrete GnRH; it is also used in fertility clinics to stimulate ovulation for the collection of eggs for in vitro fertilization.

The synthesis of oestrogen from androstenedione or testosterone involves aromatase, which is found in stromal cells of adipose tissue, mammary tumours and testicular Sertoli and Leydig cells as well as its main site in the ovary. In premenopausal women, the ovaries are the principal source of oestrogen. The synthesis of oestrogen can be inhibited with **aminoglutethimide**, which also inhibits steroidogenesis (Ch. 26). Selective aromatase inhibitors (**anastrazole**, **letrozole** and **exemestane**) are preferred as they block endogenous oestrogen synthesis leaving other steroid classes unaffected.

Antiprogestins

The glucocorticosteroid receptor antagonist RU 486 (**mifepristone**) shows antigestagenic activity and interrupts the human menstrual cycle and early pregnancy. Mifespristone acts as a partial agonist at progestogen receptors and inhibits the action of progesterone, resulting in decidual breakdown. Moreover, the actions of prostaglandins on uterine motility are accentuated, resulting in expulsion of the blastocyte. It is available for clinical use as an abortifacient and is used in combination with a prostaglandin.

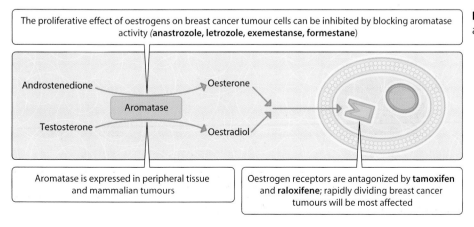

The proliferative effect of oestrogens on breast cancer tumour cells can be inhibited by blocking aromatase activity (**anastrozole, letrozole, exemestanse, formestane**)

Androstenedione

Aromatase

Testosterone

Oesterone

Oestradiol

Aromatase is expressed in peripheral tissue and mammalian tumours

Oestrogen receptors are antagonized by **tamoxifen** and **raloxifene**; rapidly dividing breast cancer tumours will be most affected

Fig. 3.27.2 Pharmacological uses for anti-oestrogens.

28. Sex hormones: male

Questions
- How is male gonadal hormone secretion regulated?
- What are the major uses for androgens and anti-androgens?

Androgens (e.g. testosterone) control spermatogenesis, sexual development, puberty and male virilization. The secretion of luteinizing hormone (referred to as interstitial cell-stimulating hormone (ICSH) in the male) and follicle-stimulating hormone (FSH) from the anterior pituitary by gonadotrophin-releasing hormone (GnRH) (Fig. 3.28.1) regulates spermatogenesis. ICSH stimulates the synthesis of testosterone by Leydig cells of the testis while FSH stimulates Sertoli cells to stimulate spermatogenesis. Testosterone acts locally to stimulate sperm production and peripherally on cells carrying testosterone receptors (steroid receptor family). The release of ICSH and FSH is regulated by testosterone, although this negative feedback mechanism becomes impaired during puberty. Testosterone is converted to its more active metabolite dihydrotestosterone by 5α-reductase, of which there are two isoforms with tissue-specific expression:

- type I: in skin, sebaceous glands, hair follicles, prostate
- type II: skin dermis and seminal vesicles, genital skin, beard and scalp hair follicles, prostate.

Type II 5α-reductase is essential for virilization of the male fetus and lack of this isoform leads to male pseudohermaphroditism. Testosterone can also be converted to oestrogens in adipose tissue by aromatase and is responsible for postmenopausal oestrogen production.

Testosterone has a variety of cellular effects within the developing male embryo (e.g. transformation of the wolffian ducts of epididymis, seminal vesicles and deferent ducts) and after puberty determines muscle mass, spermatogenesis, sexual potency, behaviour and coarsening of the voice. Dihydrotestosterone is responsible for the pubertal changes in the male and prostatic growth (Fig. 3.28.1B) and plays a role in controlling the growth of body hair (alopecia in men, hirsutism in women), enlargement of the prostate gland and acne. Both testosterone and dihydrotestosterone bind to intracellular androgen receptors, which translocate to the nucleus and alter the rate of gene transcription in Leydig cells, skeletal muscle, prostate gland, skin, sebaceous glands and brain. Mutations in the androgen receptor or in 5α-reductase result in loss of function, lack of virilization of the male embryo and pseudohermaphroditism.

Testosterone undergoes extensive first pass metabolism when administered by the oral route and is quickly absorbed from an i.m. injection. In order to improve duration of action, testosterone is administered as an ester (e.g. **cypionate**, **enanthate** and **buciclate**) by i.m. injection. The esters are hydrolysed to testosterone, which, in turn, is metabolized in the liver. Synthetic analogues, including **danazol**, **fluoxymesterone**, **methytestosterone** and **oxandrolone**, are slowly metabolized by the liver and have even longer plasma half-lives. The metabolites of these synthetic analogues are excreted in urine and faeces and, therefore, can quite easily be measured.

Pharmacological actions
A number of adverse effects are associated with the consumption of androgens by men and women. When used in women, androgens carry the risk of masculization, manifested by acne, growth of facial hair and coarsening of the voice, and menstrual irregularities, which subside following termination of androgen usage. However, long-term use is associated with male-pattern baldness, hirsutism and increased muscle mass. Androgens are best avoided in pregnancy as this will cause masculization of the female fetus. In males, androgen abuse can lead to azoospermia and gynaecomastia owing to inhibition of gonadotrophin release and conversion of androgens to oestrogen. However, this is not a side-effect seen with androgens that are poor substrates for the aromatase enzyme (e.g. **19-nortestosterone, fluoxymesterone, danzolol**). A number of other class-related side-effects from continued usage include oedema, jaundice, raised haematocrit and reduction in high density lipoproteins.

Therapeutic uses
A failure to secrete sufficient levels of testosterone will delay the onset of puberty, which is characteristic of hypogonadism. It is, however, important to ascertain that the deficiency is not caused by a failure of the hypothalamic–pituitary axis to secrete GnRH and ICSH, which is an indication of secondary hypogonadism. It is usual to treat boys with delayed puberty for periods of 4 to 6 months with testosterone. However, where testicular failure is complete, long-acting esters of testosterone (e.g. **cypionate, enanthate**) are administered i.m. for 6–12 months.

Other therapeutic uses for androgens include palliative care in breast cancer. As it has been shown that testosterone can inhibit mammary epithelial cell proliferation induced by oestrogen, addition of androgens to oestrogen replacement therapy could confer protection against the risk of breast cancer. Androgens stimulate erythropoiesis and may be of use in a variety of anaemias. Danzolol is a weak androgen but also inhibits feedback inhibition of GnRH secretion from the

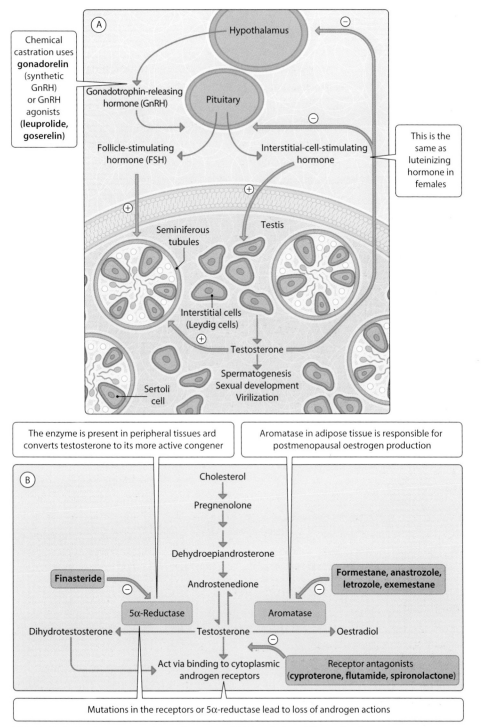

Chemical castration uses **gonadorelin** (synthetic GnRH) or GnRH agonists (**leuprolide, goserelin**)

This is the same as luteinizing hormone in females

The enzyme is present in peripheral tissues ard converts testosterone to its more active congener

Aromatase in adipose tissue is responsible for postmenopausal oestrogen production

Mutations in the receptors or 5α-reductase lead to loss of androgen actions

Fig. 3.28.1 Sex hormone release in males. (A) Regulation; (B) synthesis.

they improve performance in athletes. Steroids including nandrolone, methyltestosterone and fluoxymesterone are commonly used by body builders.

Anti-androgens

There are a number of potential sites for interference in the actions of testosterone. The synthesis of testosterone can be inhibited by reducing the amount of GnRH released from the hypothalamus and this can be achieved by continuous infusion with GnRH agonists like **leuprolide**. In these circumstances, plasma levels of ICSH and testosterone decline. **Finasteride** and **dutasteride** are selective type 2 inhibitors of 5α-reductase and inhibit the formation of dihydrotestosterone; they are used in the treatment of benign prostatic hyperplasia.

Cytoproterone acetate is a progestin derived from progesterone (17-OH-progesterone); it has anti-androgenic activity by binding to the androgen receptor, thereby inhibiting the ability of androgens to alter the rate of gene transcription; these are used in the treatment of prostatic cancer, hypersexuality and hirsutism. The non-steroidal anti-androgen **flutamide** has potent anti-androgenic activity without any glucocorticosteroid or progestogenic activity and is used in prostatic cancer. It has a short plasma half-life and is metabolized in the liver to the more active metabolite 2-hydroxyflutamide. This agent inhibits the binding of dihydrotestosterone and testosterone to their receptors. The mineralcorticosteroid antagonist **spironolactone**, which is used as a potassium-sparing diuretic, is also an androgen antagonist and can cause loss of libido and gynaecomastia.

pituitary, thereby reducing oestrogen and progestogen synthesis in the ovary. It is used to treat endometriosis, gynaecomastia and hereditary angioedema. Anabolic steroids have become notorious through their widespread use in sport in the belief

29. Non-steroidal anti-inflammatory drugs

Questions
- How are prostanoids formed and what are their actions?
- What are the major uses for NSAIDs?

Prostaglandins

Prostaglandins belong to a family of mediators known as eicosanoids, which act by both autocrine and paracrine mechanisms. Actions are short lived as they are rapidly metabolized and not stored. Chemical signals released under physiological conditions or following tissue injury stimulate target cells, triggering a rise in intracellular Ca^{2+}. This activates phospholipase A_2, which catalyses the biosynthesis of arachidonic acid from membrane phospholipids (Fig. 3.29.1). Arachidonic acid is converted to prostaglandin (PG) H_2 (an intermediary in the synthesis of prostaglandins) by cyclo-oxygenase (COX), of which there are two isoforms. COX1 is constitutively expressed and responsible for the production of prostanoids involved in important physiological actions (e.g. protecting the lining of the gastrointestinal tract from the corrosive action of gastric acid). The expression of COX2 is increased (i.e. is inducible) under inflammatory conditions through the action of cytokines on target cells. This leads to overproduction of prostaglandins, which are implicated in various conditions (e.g. rheumatoid arthritis, ankylosing spondylitis, osteoarthritis).

The pharmacological activity of prostaglandins is mediated by a number of different receptor subtypes that belong to the family of G-protein-coupled receptors with seven membrane-spanning domains and this explains their considerable biological activity (Fig. 3.29.1). For example, prostaglandins like PGI_2 and PGE_2 have cytoprotective action in the gastro-intestinal tract by stimulating bicarbonate formation, mucus secretion and blood flow to the gastric mucosa and inhibiting gastric acid secretion by parietal cells. In the kidney, prosta-glandins stimulate vasodilatation in the renal medulla and glomeruli, thereby increasing blood flow and excretion of salt and water.

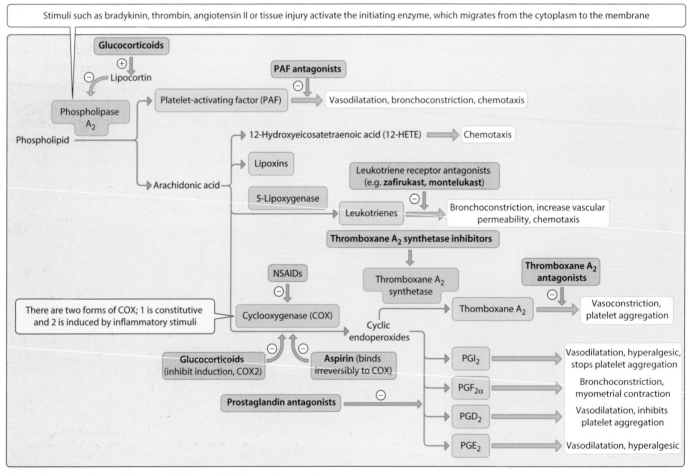

Fig. 3.29.1 Synthesis of prostaglandins and inflammatory mediators.

Pharmacological uses

There are a number of indications for the use of synthetic prostaglandin analogues. For example, **dinoprostone** (PGE_2), **carboprost tromethamine** (15-methyl $PGF_{2\alpha}$) are used as abortifacients. The intracavanosal injection of **alprostadil** (PGE_1) is used in the treatment of impotence. **Misoprostol** (oral acting analogue of PGE_1) is used in anti-ulcer treatment to protect against erosion of the stomach in patients taking NSAIDs, and **latanoprost** (analogue of $PGF_{2\alpha}$) is used to promote drainage of aqueous humour for the treatment of glaucoma.

Non-steroidal anti-inflammatory drugs

NSAIDs inhibit the formation of prostanoids by selectively targeting COX. Aspirin irreversibly inactivates COX and hence the downstream biosynthesis of prostaglandins (Fig. 3.29.2). It has a selective antiplatelet effect (inhibit TXA_2 formation) because, unlike other cells (e.g. endothelium), platelets cannot synthesize new COX and it is platelet turnover (7–10 days) that provides the only mechanism for the replenishment of functioning COX in this cell. Hence, low-dose aspirin taken on a prophylactic basis reduces the risk of stroke and myocardial infarction. Aspirin is also used to treat pain (e.g. headache), inflammation (e.g. rheumatoid arthritis) and as an antipyretic, although it does not reduce body temperature. Lipooxygenase catalyses the formation of leukotrienes, which have diverse biological activity (Fig. 3.29.1). **Montelukast** is a cysteinyl-leukotriene receptor antagonist that selectively antagonizes the biological action of leukotrienes C4 and D4 and is used in the treatment of asthma.

There are a range of structurally unrelated NSAIDs that are competitive inhibitors and do not demonstrate selectivity for COX1 and COX2. NSAIDs are used as analgesics, antipyretics and as anti-inflammatory agents; while these inhibitors have a similar mechanism of action, they differ in potency and duration of action. For example, the duration of action is short (4–8 h) for **ibuprofen**, **mefenamic acid** and **diclofenac**, intermediate (e.g. 15 h) for **naproxen** and long (24–30 h) for **phenylbutazone** and **piroxicam**. **Paracetamol** is a weak COX inhibitor and is only useful in providing analgesia and antipyresis, having poor anti-inflammatory activity.

Because NSAIDs will inhibit prostaglandins under physiological conditions, they have side-effects, the major being gastrointestinal bleeding, bronchoconstriction in some asthmatic subjects and intracerebral haemorrhage. They can cause a decline in renal function, resulting in retention of salt and water, which is exacerbated in individuals who suffer from renal impairment. Other side-effects include tinnitus (aspirin), dizziness and confusion (indometacin), and bone marrow aplasia (phenylbutazone). The last is not routinely used as an antipyretic or analgesic agent. Fatal hepatic damage can occur following acute overdose with paracetamol, which is converted to a reactive metabolite in the liver. This reactive species is normally detoxified by conjugation with glutathione but cell damage occurs if cellular levels of this protective agent are overwhelmed.

COX2-selective inhibitors (**rofecoxib**, **celecoxib**, **valdexoxib**) were developed in an attempt to reduce these untoward side-effects in patients who regularly take NSAIDs for the treatment of rheumatoid arthritis and to offer the advantage of reducing the complication of gastric bleeding frequently observed with non-selective COX inhibitors. However, recent reports show that **rofecoxib** can increase the risk of myocardial infarction in individuals who are predisposed to this condition, including the elderly and those who have previously suffered a myocardial infarction, stroke, coronary bypass or chronic heart failure. It has been withdrawn from the market.

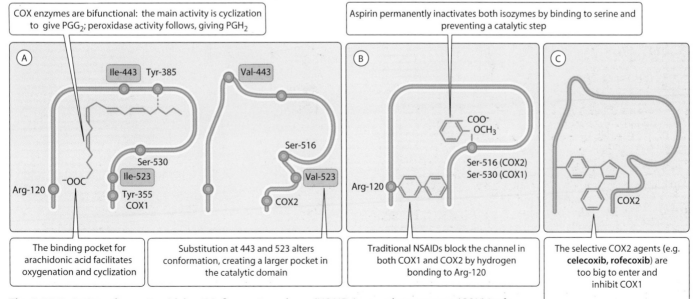

Fig. 3.29.2 Action of non-steroidal anti-inflammatory drugs (NSAIDs) on cyclooxygenase (COX) isoforms.

30. Immunomodulatory drugs

Questions
- When are immunomodulatory drugs used?
- What is the mechanism of action of immunomodulatory drugs?

The immune system has evolved to provide humoral (antibody) and cell-mediated immunity against foreign pathogens (e.g. bacteria, fungus, virus and parasites, but also foreign grafts) and malignancy (cancer); it can also act against self-antigens in pathological conditions (autoimmune disease). A variety of immunocompetent cells, including antigen-presenting cells and T and B lymphocytes, orchestrate the manner in which the body responds to a particular insult (Fig. 3.30.1). Drugs that target the immune cells are of immense benefit in the treatment of a number of diseases that involve overactivity of the immune system (Table 3.30.1) or imbalance (e.g. balance of T helper cell types affects progression of leprosy). The pharmacology of these agents in the context of rheumatoid arthritis will be used as an example.

Rheumatoid arthritis

Rheumatoid arthritis is a chronic inflammatory disease associated with swollen and painful joints, stiffness in the morning and cartilage and bone erosion. The disease is characterized by an inflamed synovial membrane, infiltration of T lymphocytes and macrophages, and deposition of rheumatoid factor and immune complexes. The production of a range of mediators, including prostaglandins, results in pain and swelling of the synovium; cytokines produced by macrophages and T lymphocytes stimulate a variety of cells (osteoclast, synoviocytes, endothelial cells) and ultimately give rise to bone and cartilage destruction. A variety of agents are used in the treatment of rheumatoid arthritis and include immunosuppressants (ciclosporin, glucocorticosteroids), the disease-modifying anti-arthritic drugs (DMARDs; gold, D-penicillamine, sulfasalazine, hydroxychloroquine and leflunomide), cytotoxic agents (azathioprine, methotrexate, cyclophosphamide) and biological agents (monoclonal antibodies against tumour necrosis factor (TNF) and interleukin (IL-1)).

Non-steroidal anti-inflammatory drugs

Non-selective (e.g. **ibuprofen**, **aspirin**, **indometacin**) and COX2-selective (e.g. **celecoxib**) NSAIDs inhibit the synthesis of prostaglandins (Ch. 29) implicated in the pain and swelling associated with rheumatoid arthritis. These drugs only provide symptomatic relief and do not prevent destruction of cartilage and bone.

Immunosuppressants

Glucocorticosteroids. Glucocorticosteroids (e.g. **prednisolone**) are effective in controlling the inflammation and may have disease-modifying effects, although they suffer from side-effects when used systemically for long periods of time (e.g. osteoporosis). Treatment with intra-articular injection of glucocorticosteroid (e.g. **triamcinolone acetonide**) can minimize these side-effects. These drugs have potent antilymphocytic action and reduce the proliferation of cells and cytokine release from lymphocytes by an action at the gene level (Ch. 26).

Ciclosporin. Ciclosporin is used to prevent transplant rejection by a selective action on T lymphocytes (Fig. 3.30.1) and this action gives it a place in the treatment of rheumatoid arthritis. Side-effects include renal insufficiency, hypertension and lymphoproliferative disease.

Disease-modifying anti-arthritic drugs

A number of drugs (**gold**, D-**penicillamine** and **sulfasalazine**) have been used for decades in the treatment of rheumatoid arthritis, while **leflunomide** is a newer agent. These are collectively known as DMARDs; however, ciclosporin and glucocorticosteroids also fall under this classification.

Cytotoxic drugs. A number of agents, including **methotrexate** (antifolate), **cyclosphosphamide** (alkylates DNA) and

Table 3.30.1 T CELLS IN DISEASE

Cell type	Normal role	Inappropriate deployment
T helper 1	Proliferation of CD8 cells, macrophages	Rheumatoid arthritis, tuberculosis, type 1 diabetes mellitus, multiple sclerosis, *Helicobacter pylori*-induced peptic ulcer
T helper 2	Response to extra-cellular antigens, driving antibody production from B cells	Allergy, asthma, schistosome infection
Cytotoxic T cells	Removal of cells with intracellular foreign protein production (malignant cells, transplant cells, viruses)	Toxic shock (over-expansion in response to bacterial endotoxins), Kawasaki disease (blood vessel inflammation)
B cells	Production of anti-bodies to foreign antigens	Autoimmune thyroiditis, agranulocytosis initiated by drugs

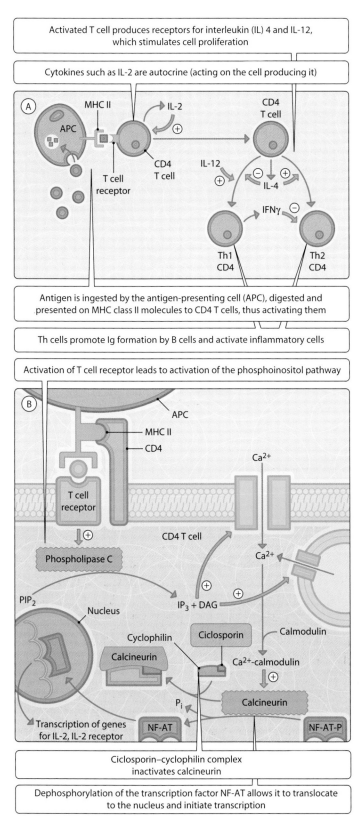

Fig. 3.30.1 Immunomodulation. (A) Activation of CD4 T cells; (B) stimulation of transcription of inflammatory mediators.

azathioprine (inhibits de novo synthesis of purines), affect both T and B cell proliferation and immune responses. Adverse effects include bone marrow suppression, liver toxicity and mutagenesis.

Gold. Gold accumulates in organs rich in phagocytic monocytes and accumulates in synovial cells. It inhibits the maturation and function of phagocytic monocytes and T cells, inhibiting phagocytic activity, and it reduces the levels of rheumatoid factor and immunoglobulins. Adverse effects of **gold sodium thiomalate** (i.m.) include lesions of the mucous membrane, which are less pronounced with **auranofin** (oral), although gastrointestinal disturbances are common. Bone marrow suppression is also observed.

D-Penicillamine. The mechanism of action of this drug is not entirely clear but its therapeutic action may be related to a reduction in the levels of rheumatoid factor. Adverse effects include leukopenia, thrombocytopenia and autoimmune syndromes.

Sulfasalazine. This drug is 5-aminosalicylic acid covalently linked to sulfapyridine; the link is cleaved by gastrointestinal bacteria. Sulfapyridine appears to reduce lymphocyte function. Adverse effects include nausea, rash, headache, hepatitis and agranulocytosis.

Hydroxychloroquine. This antimalarial agent has a number of actions that reduce macrophage and T lymphocyte function. Adverse effects include retinopathy, myopathy, rash and dermatitis.

Leflunomide. This synthetic isoxazole derivative is converted non-enzymatically in the gastrointestinal tract to an active metabolite that inhibits dihydroorotate dehydrogenase in mitochondria of immune cells. This enzyme is responsible for the synthesis of orotate, which is a precursor for the de novo synthesis of pyrimidines, important in DNA synthesis in rapidly proliferating cells. Adverse effects include diarrhoea, alopecia, liver dysfunction and teratogenicity.

Biological agents

The cytokines IL-1 and TNFα play a major role in the pathogenesis of rheumatoid arthritis. A number of biological agents targeting these cytokines have proved immensely beneficial in the treatment of this disease. These agents include **infliximab** (chimeric mouse/human) anti-TNFα monoclonal antibody, **etanercept** (genetically engineered fusion protein composed of TNF receptor and an IgG1:Fc portion) and **anakinra** (human recombinant IL-1Rα).

31. The urogenitary system

Questions
- What drugs are used in urinary incontinence and benign prostate hyperplasia?
- What drugs are used in erectile dysfunction?
- What drugs are used in the regulation of uterine motility?

Urinary incontinence

The bladder serves as a reservoir for the continual production of urine by the kidney (Fig. 3.31.1). Failure to store and empty urine appropriately gives rise to urge urinary incontinence (UUI) and stress urinary incontinence (SUI), respectively.

There is a strong desire to void in UUI as a result of an overactive bladder arising from a neurogenic dysfunction (e.g. Alzheimer's disease, Parkinson's disease, stroke and spinal cord injury). Muscarinic antagonists are used to reduce bladder contractility. **Oxybutynin** is a potent non-selective competitive muscarinic antagonist and is metabolized in the liver to the *N*-desethyl metabolite. Newer muscarinic antagonists show greater selectivity for the bladder over the salivary glands (**tolterodine, darifenacin**) and, therefore, offer better tolerability.

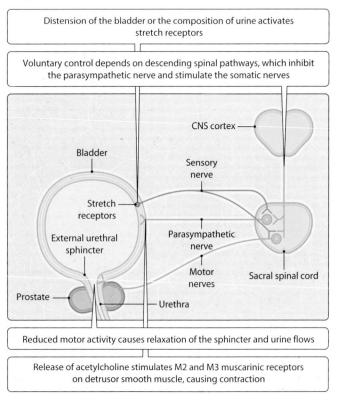

Distension of the bladder or the composition of urine activates stretch receptors

Voluntary control depends on descending spinal pathways, which inhibit the parasympathetic nerve and stimulate the somatic nerves

CNS cortex

Bladder

Sensory nerve

Stretch receptors

External urethral sphincter

Parasympathetic nerve

Motor nerves

Sacral spinal cord

Prostate

Urethra

Reduced motor activity causes relaxation of the sphincter and urine flows

Release of acetylcholine stimulates M2 and M3 muscarinic receptors on detrusor smooth muscle, causing contraction

Fig. 3.31.1 Bladder control.

In SUI, the urethral smooth muscle and sphincter are unable to generate sufficient resistance to retain urine in the bladder. The most common cause is weakness in the sphincter, which may arise from childbirth, pelvic surgery or in postmenopausal women because of a lack of oestrogen. In men, it can arise following prostate surgery. Norepinephrine from sympathetic nerves innervating urethral smooth muscle activates a number of α-adrenoceptor subtypes including α_{1A}-, α_{1B}- and α_{1D}-adrenoceptors, thereby contracting smooth muscle and increasing resistance, which reduces the flow of urine.

Midodrine (Portugal and Finland) and **phenylpropanolamine** (USA) are non-selective α-agonists and have limited usefulness because of a lack of selectivity for the bladder, with potential for unacceptable increase in blood pressure. An alternative approach is to enhance the activity of serotonin pathways within the CNS, which is known to exert an inhibitory action on parasympathetic input to the bladder and thereby reduce voiding. **Duloxetine** a specific inhibitor of serotonin and norepinephrine uptake, increases the activation of $5HT_{1A}$ inhibitory pathways, thereby reducing voiding. A peripheral mechanism may also contribute toward the effects of this drug by preventing reuptake of norepinephrine in the bladder and thereby increasing the concentration of norepinephrine at neuroeffector sites in urethral smooth muscle and increasing urethral pressure.

Benign prostatic hyperplasia

The prostate surrounds the urethra below the bladder and supplies fluid for sperm that has collected in the seminal vesicles. Hyperplasia of the prostate can lead to enlargement, which may not cause any urethral obstruction. When it does, symptoms include increased voiding frequency (common at night), difficulty in voiding and increased urge of voiding. Non-selective α_1-adrenoceptor antagonists (**tamsulosin, doxazosin, terazosin** and **alfuzosin**), induce relaxation of the urethral smooth muscle, resulting in increased urinary flow. They may also promote apoptosis in the prostate, which would reduce the size of the gland. Postural hypotension is one of the side-effects of these drugs and is caused by antagonism of α-adrenoceptors in vascular smooth muscle. The 5α-reductase inhibitors (**finasteride, dutasteride**), which block the conversion of testosterone to the more active dihydrotestosterone, have also found a place in the treatment of benign prostatic hyperplasia; their use causes atrophy of the prostatic epithelium, thereby reducing gland size. Side-effects from treatment include erectile dysfunction, altered libido, ejaculatory disorders and gynaecomastia.

Male erectile dysfunction

The inability to maintain or develop an erection during sexual stimulation is associated with ageing and diseases such as hypertension, diabetes, cardiovascular disease, depression and neurological conditions. Blood flow into the flaccid penis is impeded by contraction of vascular smooth muscle while increased blood flow to the corpus cavernosum following vaso-dilatation of blood vessels and excitation of cavernosal smooth muscle cells leads to an erection. Sexual stimulation triggers the activation of nitrergic nerves and release of nitric oxide (NO), raising intracellular cGMP and culminating in relaxation of smooth muscle and filling of the sinusoidal spaces of the carvernosum (Fig. 3.31.2B). Pharmacological approaches include **sildenafil**, **tadalafil** and **vardenafil**, which are potent inhibitors of phosphodiesterase (PDE) 5 and prevent the inactivation of cGMP. Sildenafil also inhibits PDE6, which is present in retinal cells, leading to visual disturbances (blue vision). As these agents increase the actions of NO, they should not be administered to patients taking nitrovasodilator drugs or with cardiovascular disease.

Prostaglandins (PGE$_2$) are synthesized by the corpus cavernosum endothelium and smooth muscle and may play a role in erectile function. The intracavernosal injection or urethral application of PGE$_1$ (**alprostadil**) causes an erection.

Side-effects of repeated injection can include priapism, scar formation, burning sensations and lightheadedness. The non-selective dopamine receptor agonist **apomorphine** acts centrally to increase blood flow in the prefrontal cortex, and neurons within this region activate nitrergic nerves in the corpus cavernosum; this drug is licensed in Europe and Japan.

Uterine motility

There are a number of pharmacological agents that either stimulate (oxytocic) or suppress (tocolytic: terbutaline, ritodrine, magnesium sulphate, nifedipine are used in premature labour) uterine contraction (Fig. 3.31.2C). **Oxytocin** is usually the drug of choice for the induction of labour and is administered i.v. The uterus is extremely sensitive to the excitatory action of oxytocin and care must be taken when using this agent. In certain circumstances, tocolytics may be required to suppress overstimulation of the uterus as this can reduce placental circulation. Following birth, the administration of ergot alkaloids (**ergonovine**, **methyergonovine**) and prostglandins (**alprostadil** (PGE$_1$), **dinoprostone** (PGE$_2$), **carboprost** (15-methyl-PGF$_{2\alpha}$)) greatly reduces the risk of postpartum haemorrhage. Ergot alkaloids are administered orally while prostanoids are administered by i.m., intra-amniotic or intravaginal routes.

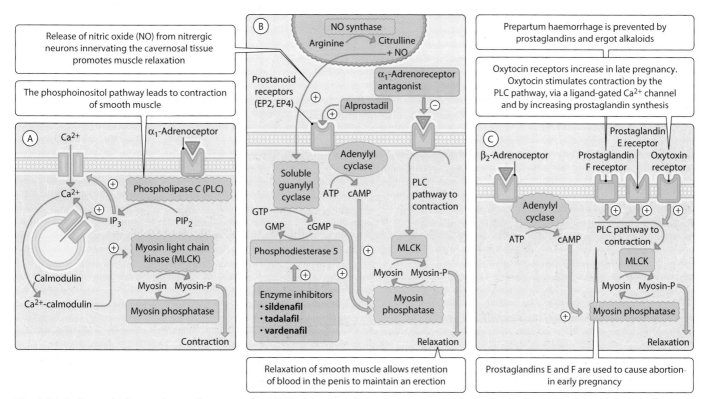

Fig. 3.31.2 Control of smooth muscle contraction. (A) Pathway leading to contraction; (B) erectile dysfunction; (C) modulation of uterine motility.

32. The eye

Questions
- How does the autonomic system regulate pupil size?
- What drugs are used in the treatment of glaucoma?

Pupil size is controlled by light and the activity of the parasympathetic and sympathetic nervous systems. The release of acetylcholine from parasympathetic nerves contracts the circular smooth muscle of the iris, resulting in pupil constriction (miosis). In contrast, norepinephrine released from sympathetic nerves innervating radial smooth muscle stimulates pupil dilatation. Contraction of ciliary smooth muscle initiated by acetylcholine relieves tension in suspensory ligaments and the lens adopts a spherical shape. This allows the lens to accommodate for near vision. Contraction of ciliary smooth muscle also promotes drainage of aqueous humour through the trabecular network and via the canal of Schlemm (Fig. 3.32.1). Occlusion of the outflow channels impaires and outflow of aqueous humour from the anterior chamber increases intraocular pressure (glaucoma). This increase can lead to degeneration of the retinal ganglion cells, visual impairment and blindness. Primary open-angle glaucoma is the most common form and is associated with structural changes to the trabecular network leading to increased resistance to drainage of aqueous humour, which can be treated pharmacologically. Acute-angle closure is a sudden obstruction of the angle of the anterior chamber by the iris and may occur in structurally predisposed eyes, in which the angle of the anterior chamber is narrow, or as a result of a mature cataract, dilatation of the eye (in dim light), stimulation of the sympathetic nervous system or anticholinergic drugs. Treatment to reduce intraocular pressure involves peripheral laser iridectomy or surgical iridectomy.

Agents used for diagnostic purposes
The retinal surface can be inspected easily by inducing pupil dilatation (mydriasis) and paralysis of the ciliary body (cycloplegia). Muscarinic antagonists including **tropicamide** have relatively short duration (3 h) while **cyclopentolate** and **homatropine** have considerably longer duration of action (24 h). The α_1-adrenoceptor agonists produce a weak mydriatic action without cycloplegia (**phenylephrine**).

Glaucoma
A variety of pharmacological agents are used to decrease the production of aqueous humour or to increase its outflow from the conventional (canal of Schlemm) or uveoscleral pathway.

Inhibition of aqueous humour formation
The β-adrenoceptor antagonists (**timolol** and **betaxolol**) are the first-line treatment for glaucoma; applied topically to the eye, they inhibit production of aqueous humour by the ciliary epithelium and reduce intraocular pressure (Fig. 3.32.1C). Their use is contraindicated in patients with asthma. The production of aqueous humour can also be inhibited by α_2-adrenoceptor agonists such as **apraclonidine** and **brimonidine** (highly selective), which are thought to have a direct action on α_2-adrenoceptors on the ciliary epithelium and an indirect action via presynaptic inhibition of norepinephrine release from sympathetic neurons. **Dipivefrin** is a prodrug of epinephrine and is rapidly metabolized by esterases within the aqueous humour; it acts indirectly by inducing vasoconstriction and reducing blood flow in the ciliary body, thereby reducing aqueous humour formation. Being a mydriatic, this agent is contraindicated in patients with acute-angle glaucoma. It can be combined with a β-adrenoceptor antagonist.

Carbonic anhydrase is involved in the formation of aqueous humour, producing bicarbonate from water and carbon dioxide within epithelial cells of the ciliary body. The enzyme is inhibited by **acetazolamide** (oral) but this drug suffers from a number of side-effects through its inhibition of carbonic anhydrase at other sites (e.g. loss of taste, gastritis and metabolic acidosis). **Dorzolamide** is applied topically and and is better tolerated by patients.

Promoting aqueous humour outflow
Aqueous humour outflow can be enhanced by the muscarinic agonist **pilocarpine**, which stimulates ciliary smooth muscle contraction, thus opening the trabecular network and decreasing resistance to outflow (Fig. 3.32.1C). An undesirable effect is miosis and accommodative spasm, which reduces the amount of light entering the eye and the field of vision; patients taking this drug are not advised to drive. Indirect acting parasympathomimetic agents, such as the acetylcholinesterase inhibitors **demecarium bromide** and **echothiopate iodide**, are rarely used. A number of ester prodrug derivatives of prostaglandin $F_{2\alpha}$ (**latanoprost**, **travoprost** and **unoprostone**) stimulate FP receptors in the ciliary body and enhance the outflow of fluid from the uveoscleral route. **Bimatoprost** is an amide derivative that appears to be resistant to hydrolysis and can act directly on the receptor. Side-effects of this drug class include increase in iris pigmentation, increased length and thickness of the eyelash and pigmentation of the skin of the eyelids.

Allergic disease

Allergic conjunctivitis is caused by direct exposure of the eye to airborne allergens and is the most common hypersensitivity reaction in the eye. Swelling, lacrimation, itching, soreness and redness are unwanted effects triggered by mast cell-derived histamine. Hence, topical application of antihistamines (**levocabastine**, **emedastine**, **azelastine** and **antazoline**) or mast cell-stabilizing agents (**lodoxamide**, **nedocromil sodium**, **sodium cromoglicate**) is clinically efficacious. Topical gluco-corticosteroids are also used for short-term treatment of allergic disease in the eye but are associated with unwanted ocular side-effects including increased ocular pressure and cataract formation. However, modified steroids including **loteprodnel** and **rimexolone**, which undergo rapid inactivation in the anterior chamber, are of use in acute and chronic treatment of allergic conjunctivitis. Glucocorticosteroids are also used in the treatment of keratitis and uveitis.

Infections

Superficial ocular bacterial infections (e.g. bacterial conjunctivitis, blepharitis, keratitis and styes) or internal infections (e.g. endophthalmitis) are commonplace. Fluoroquinolones (e.g. **ciprofloxacin**, **olfoxacin**, **lomefloxacin**, **moxifloxacin** and **gatifloxacin**) represent the latest in a long line of broad-spectrum antibiotics. In viral infections, **aciclovir** (oral) or **trifluridine** and **vidarabine** (topical) are used in the treatment of herpes simplex infection (causing epithelial and stromal keratitis) and **ganciclovir** for the treatment of cytomegalovirus infection, particularly in patients with HIV.

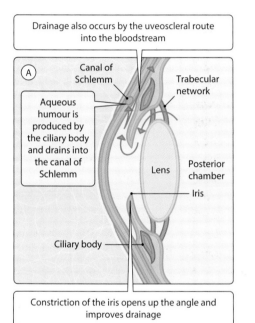

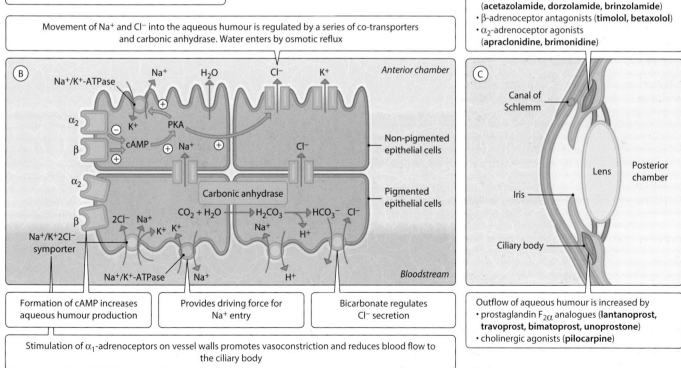

Fig. 3.32.1 The eye and aqueous humour. (A) Drainage; (B) formation of aqueous humour; (C) drugs used in glaucoma.

33. The skin

Questions
- What is the pathology of acne, psoriasis and dermatitis?
- What drugs are used in the treatment of these diseases?

The skin is an important barrier to the external environment, a sensory organ (touch, heat, cold) and regulates body temperature (sweating). Non-allergic and allergic inflammatory conditions lead to disruption in this function and are a common cause of morbidity (e.g. acne, psoriasis, dermatitis). By its very nature, the skin is amenable to topical application of pharmacological agents (e.g. ointments, pastes, lotions and creams).

Acne

Acne is a condition of the hair follicles involving excessive sebum production, bacterial infection (*Propionibacterium acnes*), desquamation of follicular epithelium and inflammation (Fig. 3.33.1A). A number of topical treatments are available.

Benzoyl peroxide. This is a frequently used first-line therapy and has strong antibacterial activity, reducing colonization by *P. acnes*. Benzoyl peroxide causes drying and skin irritation and contact allergy may develop in susceptible individuals.

Salicylic acid. This is a keratolytic agent that breaks down follicular plugs and the rate of follicular desquamation, thereby reducing the number of comedones. It may exacerbate inflammatory acne lesions through erythema and peeling.

Azelaic acid. This naturally occurring dicarboxylic acid inhibits DNA synthesis in keratinocytes and is reported to have a comedolytic activity. It is mildly irritating and can cause skin lightening in dark-skinned individuals.

Topical antibiotics. Antibiotics are used to reduce the number of bacteria in the pilosebaceous duct and have a mild comedolytic effect. They are administered orally in patients with severe acne or when topical therapy fails. Examples of antibiotics used for the treatment of acne include the tetracyclines (**tetracycline, minocycline, doxycycline, lymecycline**), **erythromycin**, **clindamycin** and **cotrimoxazole**. Side-effects from oral administration include gastrointestinal disturbances, vaginal candidiasis, pseudomembranous colitis, sensitization of skin to sunlight and bacterial resistance.

Topical retinoids. Derivatives of vitamin A (retinol), including **tretinoin** and **isotretinoin**, bind to retinoic acid receptors (RAR). These receptors regulate gene transcription critical for cell proliferation and differentiation and are used in non-inflammatory and inflammatory acne lesions. They are effective comedolytic agents and normalize the desquamation of follicular epithelium and minimize the inflammatory response. Newer analogues include **adapalene** and **tazarotene**. Adapalene has less irritant action compared with tretinoin. In severe acne, oral administration of retinoids (isotretinoin) is highly effective. Retinoids are teratogenic and contraception is highly advisable in women; hypertriglyceridaemia and hypercholesterolaemia occur.

Psoriasis

Psoriasis is a chronic disease that affects the skin and joints and is characterized by rapid proliferation of the epidermis, resulting in scaling erythematous plaques. The psoriatic lesion is characterized by increased proliferation of keratinocytes (plaques), increased vascularization and presence of activated inflammatory cells. A variety of cytokines secreted from lymphocytes, dendritic cells and keratinocytes (e.g. interferon-γ, interleukins 1β and 8 and tumour necrosis factor-α) amplify and perpetuate these changes. Treatment strategies are designed to inhibit epidermal cell proliferation and inflammation (Fig. 3.33.1B). Topical therapy includes tars (coal, wood), isotretinoin, tazarotene (retinoids) and anthralin. Oral therapy includes retinoids (acitretin), **psoralens** (PUVA: psoralen plus ultraviolet A), **ciclosporin** (suppresses cell-mediated immune responses) and **methotrexate** (inhibits dihydrofolate reductase, thereby inhibiting DNA synthesis).

Tars (e.g. wood, coal) and anthralin (anthrones). These are applied to the skin then removed after a defined period of time and the affected area exposed to ultraviolet light (UVB). The mechanism of action is not clear but the appearance of plaques is reduced. Skin irritation and staining occurs.

Vitamin D analogues. **Calcipotriene** and **tacalcitol** are applied topically. They bind to nuclear receptors of the thyroid and retinoid receptor family. The receptors for vitamin D are found in epidermal keratinocytes, dermal fibroblasts, antigen-presenting cells and lymphocytes. The activation of vitamin D-response elements in specific genes inhibits keratinocyte proliferation, induces keratinocyte differentiation and has anti-inflammatory activity. Side-effects include local irritation and in rare cases hypercalcaemia.

Retinoids. Topical retinoids (e.g. **tazarotene**) may promote terminal differentiation of keratinocytes and may interfere with cytokine production by inflammatory cells. Side-effects include dryness of the mucous membranes and burning sensation in the skin. **Acitretin** is an orally available retinoid used in the treatment of psoriasis and is the active metabolite of the prodrug **etretinate**. Both are teratogenic and pregnancy must be avoided in women taking these agents. Use as either monotherapy or combined with phototherapy has proved effective.

Phototherapy. Phototherapy with UVB (narrowband: 311 nm) or photochemotherapy with UVA (320–400 nm plus photo-sensitizing psorlanes) are highly effective in the treatment of psoriasis. Psoralens (**methoxsalen**, **trioxsalen**) are orally bioavailable and intercalate with DNA following UVA irradiation of the skin. The cross-linking of psoralen with DNA prevents proliferation of cells. Narrow-band UVB treatment offers the advantage that no photosensitizing agent is required. Side-effects of PUVA treatment include nausea and blistering. In situations where phototherapy does not adequately treat patients, then a number of systemic agents can be employed including methotrexate and ciclosporin (Ch. 31).

Dermatitis

Dermatitis may be caused by contact with an irritant (e.g. acids, alkalis, solvents) or contact with sensitizing agents such as metals in jewellery (e.g. nickel), toxic substances in plants (e.g. poison ivy), rubber (latex) and antibiotics. Atopic dermatitis occurs in individuals with a familial history of allergy and is prevalent in children. There is inflammation of the upper layers of the skin, resulting in itching, blisters, redness, swelling and scaling (Fig. 3.33.1C). Damage to the skin by uncontrolled scratching can lead to bacterial infection. Topical administration of **glucocorticosteroids** has a number of beneficial actions in dermatitis: prevents formation of prostanoids and leukotrienes; induces apoptosis of eosinophils; decreases eosinophil, lymphocyte, monocyte and tissue mast cell number; decreases expression of adhesion molecules on vascular endothelium; inhibits transcription of proinflammatory cytokines (e.g. interferon-γ, interleukins 4 and 5 and tumour necrosis factor-α); reduces keratinocyte proliferation; and causes vasoconstriction. Severe atopic dermatitis is treated with **ciclosporin**, **azathioprine** (cytotoxic immunosuppressant affecting purine metabolism and altering the synthesis of RNA and DNA) and **methotrexate**. Pruritis (itch) can be controlled with sedating, centrally active H₁ antagonists (e.g. diphenhydramine) and by non-sedating peripherally acting drugs (e.g. loratidine). Cetirizine has anti-inflammatory and antihistamine actions and is, therefore, of some utility in this disease.

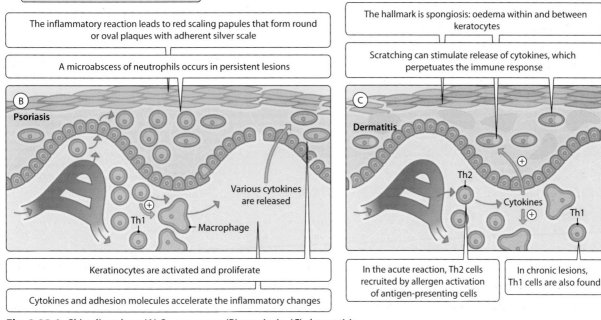

Fig. 3.33.1 Skin disorders. (A) Severe acne; (B) psoriasis; (C) dermatitis.

34. Parkinson's disease

Questions
■ What is the pathology of Parkinson's disease?
■ What drugs are used in its treatment?

Parkinson's disease is a neurodegenerative disorder that involves selective destruction of dopaminergic neurons in the basal ganglia (Fig. 3.34.1), resulting in abnormalities of motor function including bradykinesia (slow movement), rigidity, resting tremor and disturbances in gait. These symptoms can be ameliorated by therapeutic intervention (Fig. 3.34.2); however, the neurodegeneration is not reversed.

Drug treatments

Levodopa
Dopamine is synthesized in nigrostriatal neurons from the precursor levodopa by aromatic amino acid decarboxylase (dopa decarboxylase). Degeneration of dopaminergic neurons reduces dopamine levels, which can be restored with levodopa. Levodopa is administered orally and extensively metabolized to dopamine by dopa decarboxylase and to 3-O-methyldopa by the enzyme catechol-O-methyltransferase (COMT) in the periphery. Levodopa, unlike dopamine, is transported into the CNS where it is converted to dopamine, stored and released in presynaptic neurons within the nigrostriatal region.

The unwanted side-effects of levodopa result from its conversion to dopamine in the periphery. These include nausea, vomiting (stimulation of chemoreceptor trigger zone) and hypotension. These can be minimized by coadministration with a decarboxylase inhibitor (**carbidopa** or **benserazide**) that does not cross the blood–brain barrier and, therefore, prevents the conversion of levodopa to dopamine selectively in the periphery. Consequently, a lower dose of levodopa can then be administered to achieve the desired therapeutic effect. The administration of a dopamine antagonist (**domperidone**) that does not cross the blood–brain barrier can also be used to reduce the peripheral side-effects associated with levodopa.

The beneficial effects of levodopa declines because the capacity of the nigrostriatal dopaminergic neurons to store and release dopamine declines as neurodegeneration progresses ('wearing off' or 'end of dose deterioration'). Patients also develop excessive movements (dyskinesia) with prolonged use of levodopa that appear when levodopa plasma concentration is low (the 'on/off' phenomenon). Under physiological conditions, nigrostriatal neurons release dopamine tonically in a continuous manner, resulting in persistent stimulation of post-

synaptic dopamine receptors. The administration of levodopa in patients leads to a pulsatile release of dopamine. It is this intermittent stimulation of postsynaptic receptors that is thought to underlie dyskinesia. This unwanted effect can be delayed with the use of dopamine agonists.

Dopamine agonists
An alternative to levodopa is the use of dopamine agonists, which offer a number of advantages. Dopamine agonists act directly on dopamine receptors on GABAergic neurons in the striatum and so neurodegeneration of dopaminergic neurons does not limit their effects. Levodopa is non-selective ($D_{1–5}$), while dopamine agonists selective for D_1 and D_2 receptors can minimize the potential for side-effects. The dopamine receptor agonists have considerably longer duration of action than dopamine and, therefore, stimulation of receptors is more

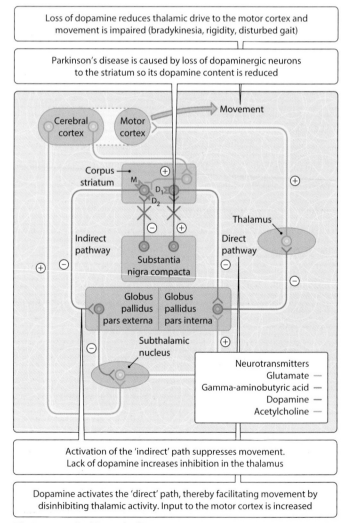

Loss of dopamine reduces thalamic drive to the motor cortex and movement is impaired (bradykinesia, rigidity, disturbed gait)

Parkinson's disease is caused by loss of dopaminergic neurons to the striatum so its dopamine content is reduced

Activation of the 'indirect' path suppresses movement. Lack of dopamine increases inhibition in the thalamus

Dopamine activates the 'direct' path, thereby facilitating movement by disinhibiting thalamic activity. Input to the motor cortex is increased

Fig. 3.34.1 Parkinson's disease.

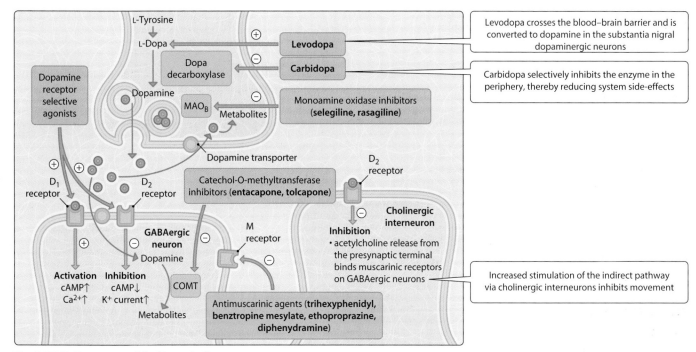

Fig. 3.34.2 Treatment of Parkinson's disease.

persistent than pulsatile and dyskinesia is less of a problem. Finally, the metabolism of dopamine in nigrostriatal neurons can produce oxygen radicals, which may contribute to neurodegeneration. This would not be observed with dopamine agonists. Side-effects include hypotension, which in rare cases may be profound after the initial dose. Insomnia and confusion similar to those observed in schizophrenia may occur and are attributed to dopaminergic overactivity within the CNS. Other adverse effects include constipation, peripheral vasospasm (agonists are structurally related to ergot alkaloids) and nausea.

Monoamine oxidase inhibitors
Dopamine is taken up into dopaminergic neurons and undergoes oxidative metabolism by monoamine oxidase (MAO) of which there are two isoforms: MAOA is located predominantly, but not exclusively, in the periphery while MAOB is found centrally. **Selegiline** is a selective MAOB inhibitor and, therefore, prolongs the duration of action of dopamine released from nigrostriatal neurons and reduces the potential for 'wearing off' and the 'on/off' phenomenon. Another potential benefit of inhibiting dopamine metabolism is the reduction of oxygen radical production, and, therefore, the use of MAOB inhibitors in the early stages of the disease may reduce neurodegeneration of nigrostriatal neurons. Non-selective MAO inhibitors (e.g. **isocarboxazid**) will potentiate the actions of catecholamines in the periphery (e.g. vasoconstriction: throbbing headache and hypertension) and so the consumption of foods and beverages high in tyramine content (e.g. wine, cheese) should be avoided as it potentiates the sympathomimetic actions of this agent. This is not observed with selegiline, although metabolites of selegiline include amphetamine, which can induce anxiety and insomnia.

Catechol-O-methyltransferase inhibitors
The bioavailability of levodopa can be increased by inhibiting conversion of dopamine to the inactive metabolites 3,4-dihydroxyphenyl acetic acid and 3-methoxytyramine. Examples of COMT inhibitors include **entacapone** and **tolcapone**; the latter crosses the blood–brain barrier. Side-effects include nausea, diarrhoea and hepatoxicity (tolcapone).

Anticholinergic agents
Excitatory cholinergic interneurons within the striatum activate GABAergic neurons. The loss of dopaminergic neurons can lead to overactivation of cholinergic neurons and persistent stimulation of GABAergic neurons. Muscarinic antagonists (benztropine) inhibit the postsynaptic activation of these neurons. They are less effective than levodopa against tremor and rigidity but reduce the excessive salivation in some patients; they have little effect on bradykinesia.

Amantadine
Originally introduced as an antiviral drug, amantadine has proven to be of some clinical use in Parkinson's disease. It stimulates the release of stored dopamine and reduces reuptake into nerve terminals. Its pharmacological activity relies on the presence of dopaminergic neurons, so it is given during the early stages of the disease. Side-effects include ankle swelling, confusion at high doses and vasoconstriction of the skin through local catecholamine release (livedo reticularis).

35. Anxiolytics, sedatives and hypnotics

Questions
- What are the characteristic features of anxiety?
- What drugs are used in the treatment of anxiety?

Anxiety is a condition associated with excessive excitatory neurotransmission in the CNS that clinically is characterized by nervousness and apprehension concerning a variety of activities or events and is a reaction to stress or altered circumstances (e.g. bereavement). It is also associated with a state of sympathetic arousal (e.g. palpitations, sweating, headache and restlessness). The manifestation of anxiety is a result of a complex interaction between different brain structures (Fig. 3.35.1). A number of neuronal pathways, involving GABA, serotonin (5HT) and norepinephrine are implicated in modulating anxiety and provide a rational basis for treatment.

Benzodiazepines
Gamma-aminobutyric acid (GABA) is the major inhibitory neurotransmitter in the CNS and activates ionotropic $GABA_A$ receptors on postsynaptic neurons (Fig. 3.35.2). The overstimulation of these receptors can result in sedation, amnesia and ataxia, while insufficient stimulation can lead to arousal, anxiety, insomnia and seizures. $GABA_A$ receptors are multimeric complexes that gate the movement of Cl^- into neurons, evoking fast inhibitory synaptic potentials and reducing neuronal excitability in postsynaptic neurons. Benzodiazepines bind to a regulatory site (α-subunit) on the $GABA_A$ receptor that is distinct from the GABA-binding site (β-subunit) and increase the frequency of channel opening, thereby enhancing the inhibitory actions of GABA throughout the CNS (e.g. cortex, hippocampus and amygdala).

Benzodiazepines are used for short-term treatment of severe anxiety, insomnia (hypnotics), epilepsy, acute alcohol withdrawal and preoperative sedation. They are being increasingly replaced with selective serotonin reuptake inhibitors (SSRIs) for the treatment of anxiety, as these are safer. Long-term use of benzodiazepines as sleeping pills is best avoided because of undesirable effects. The benzodiazapines are orally bioavailable. **Diazepam** is converted to active metabolites in the liver (e.g. *N*-desmethyldiazepam), which have a considerably longer duration of action. In contrast, **lorazepam** and **alprazolam** are more rapidly inactivated and have shorter plasma half-lives. Benzodiazepines may be administered i.v. for the emergency treatment of epilepsy (diazepam) or as a premedication for surgery (midazolam).

This drug class is associated with a number of important adverse effects. Drowsiness and impaired motor coordination are important side-effects, particularly if patients need to drive or operate machinery. Overdose with benzodiazepines alone will prolong sleep but does not lead to respiratory or CNS depression, although the effects can be life threatening if administered in combination with alcohol, barbiturates or antihistamines. The $GABA_A$ receptor antagonist **flumazenil** can be useful in acute overdose but can cause seizures.

The major shortcomings of benzodiazepines are hangover, tolerance and drug dependence; the mechanism of these effects is not entirely known but will involve adaptive changes within the CNS. Tolerance develops with chronic use and, therefore, short-term treatment is advisable. Tolerance to the sedative effects of these drugs may be beneficial when treating anxiety. Drug dependence, is a major problem and cessation can give rise to rebound anxiety, tremor, insomnia and loss of appetite. These symptoms appear more slowly with benzodiazepines with long plasma half-life and more abruptly with the shorter-duration benzodiazepines.

Non-benzodiazepine drugs
Zopiclone, **zolpidem** and **zaleplon** are non-benzodiazepine sedative/hypnotic drugs used for short-term treatment of

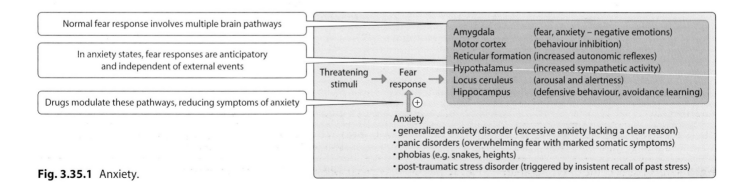

Fig. 3.35.1 Anxiety.

insomnia. They display high affinity for GABA$_A$ receptors containing the α_1-subunit and mutational studies suggest that this subunit is responsible for the sedative and anticonvulsant properties of benzodiazepines, while anxiolysis is associated with the $\alpha_{2/3}$-subunits. Hence, there is the potential for developing non-sedative anxiolytic drugs targeting GABA$_A$ receptors.

The short duration (half-life) of action (zaleplon, 1 h; zolpidem, 2.5 h; zopiclone, 5 h) explains their limited hangover effect and development of tolerance but dependence can occur. These drugs should not be used for periods of longer than 4 weeks and are unsuitable as anxiolytic or anticonvulsant drugs.

Drugs affecting serotonergic neurotransmission

Azapirones.   Drugs commonly used to treat depression have also been useful in anxiety disorders. The role of serotonergic and noradrenergic pathways in anxiety (Fig. 3.35.1) provides a rationale for the use of azapirones and antidepressant agents (see below). **Buspirone** has no action on GABA$_A$ receptors but is a partial 5HT$_{1A}$ receptor agonist and has anxiolytic activity. It is useful in generalized anxiety disorders but is without the attendant sedative or muscle relaxant actions characteristic of benzodiazepines. 5HT$_{1A}$ receptors are present on dorsal raphe neurons and receptor activation decreases firing of raphe serotonergic neurons (Fig. 3.35.3). Unlike benzodiazepines, which are effective after a single dose, there is a lag of approximately 2 weeks before any clinical benefit is observed. It has been suggested that reduced firing of the raphe nuclei may not fully explain

the anxiolytic action of this agent and a more complex effect on postsynaptic serotonin receptors cannot be excluded. Side-effects include gastrointestinal disturbances, dizziness and headache. The azapirones do not cause sedation, tolerance, dependence, anticonvulsant activity or cross-tolerance with alcohol, and there is no evidence of withdrawal following abrupt discontinuation.

Antidepressants.   Some antidepressants are also effective in various generalized anxiety disorders. Monoamine oxidase inhibitors (**phenelzine**, **moclobemide**), selective serotonin reuptake inhibitors (SSRIs; **citalopram**, **paroxetine**, **fluoxetine**, **sertraline**), serotonin/norepinephrine reuptake inhibitor (**venlafaxine**) and tricyclic antidepressants (**doxepin**, **clomipramine**) regulate serotonin and/or norepinephrine in the brain. SSRIs are increasingly being used for anxiety disorders because they lack the addictive properties of benzodiazepines. However, improvement in symptoms requires up to 6 weeks of treatment and most likely involves compensatory changes in neuronal circuitry in the brain. SSRIs elevate serotonin levels within the vicinity of pre- and postsynaptic receptors and this indirectly results in anxiolysis.

Beta-blockers

Anxiety is often associated with overactivation of the sympathetic nervous system, manifested in symptoms such as sweating, tremor, palpitations and diarrhoea, which can arise during social situations. **Propranolol** and **atenolol** antagonize the peripheral actions of norepinephrine and epinephrine, thereby reducing the physiological response to activation of the sympathetic nervous system.

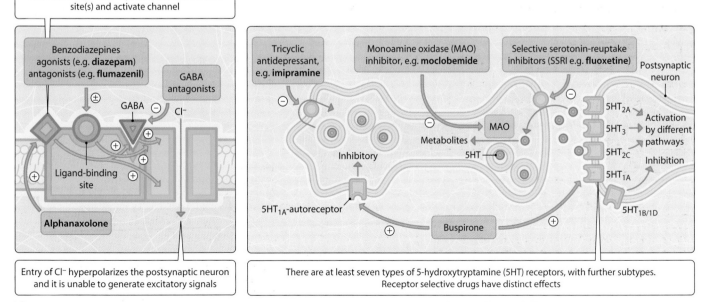

Fig. 3.35.2 Control of the GABA$_A$ receptor.   **Fig. 3.35.3** Drugs acting on serotonergic neurotransmission.

36. Antidepressants

Questions
- What are the characteristic features of depression?
- What drugs are used in the treatment of depression?

Clinical manifestation of depression is one of misery, a loss of enjoyment or participation in activities, sleep disturbances, loss of appetite and anxiety. The patient is pessimistic, lacks, self confidence, feels hopelessness, and may have suicidal tendencies. The intensity of these symptoms is increased in severe depression and the patient may suffer from hallucinations or become delusional. In less severe depression, the symptoms may be of a lesser intensity and are best described as neurotic (e.g. obsessional symptoms). In mania, subjects may exhibit hyperexcitable states, the seeming opposite of depression. Hence, affective disorders may be classified as either unipolar (mania or depression) or bipolar (both). The historical observation that patients treated with reserpine, which depletes sympathetic neurons of norepinephrine stores, suffered induced depression while patients treated with the antituberculosis drug isoniazid (shown to inhibit monoamine oxidase (MAO)) experienced relieved depression formed the rationale for developing drugs that elevate biogenic amines (serotonin, norepinephrine) within the CNS to treat depression. A complex interaction between several brain regions, serotonergic and noradrenergic nerves is implicated in depression (Fig. 3.36.1). Clinical benefits take weeks to manifest for a range of antidepressants indicating that a resetting of the activity of these neural circuits is required, rather than simply elevating neurotransmitter levels at synapses.

Monoamine oxidase inhibitors

MAO metabolizes the biogenic amines and occurs in two isoforms, both metabolizing dopamine. MAOA metabolizes serotonin and norepinephrine outside storage vesicles, thus increasing the building blocks for new neurotransmitter synthesis into synaptic vesicles (Fig. 3.36.2). MAOB is selective for phenylethylamine.

Some MAO inhibitors are non-selective (e.g. **phenelzine** and **tranylcypromine**) and patients who are prescribed these agents should refrain from consuming food and drink high in tyramine (e.g. cheese, wine) or medications such as nasal decongestants as these drugs will also augment sympathetic activity at peripheral terminals in response to tyramine (indirectly releases norepinephrine). Side-effects include dry mouth, tremor, blurred vision, throbbing headache, hypertension and CNS stimulation. More selective and reversible inhibitors of MAOA (e.g. **moclobemide**, **brofaromine**, **toloxatone** and **cimoxatone**) have more tolerable side-effects and are used for depression.

Tricyclic antidepressants

Tricyclic antidepressants (TCAs, e.g. **amitriptyline**, **imipramine**, **doxepin**, **chlomipramine**, **nortriptyline** and **desipramine**) inhibit monamine uptake in serotonergic and noradrenergic neurons, thereby increasing the concentration of these biogenic amines at synaptic sites (Fig. 3.36.2). These agents also block a number of receptor subtypes, which accounts for their side-effects, including postural hypotension (α_1), sedation (H_1), dry mouth, blurred vision and constipation (antimuscarinic). One peripheral side-effect is increased norepinephrine in the heart, resulting in heart block and arrhythmias in overdose.

Selective reuptake inhibitors

Selective serotonin reuptake inhibitors (SSRI). These are the most commonly used drugs in the treatment of depression (e.g. **fluoxetine**, **paroxetine**, **citalopram**) and selectively block the transport of serotonin into serotonergic neurons and have considerably lower affinity for a number of G-protein-coupled receptors compared with TCAs and MAO inhibitors; consequently, they have a better safety profile. Side-effects are related to the increase in availability of 5HT at postsynaptic receptor sites within the CNS and peripheral tissue. These include nausea, diarrhoea, anxiety, panic attacks, insomnia and sexual dysfunction. Sudden discontinuation of SSRIs may result in withdrawal symptoms including anxiety, irritability and dizziness. They have no anticholinergic, cardiotoxic effect or toxicity in overdose

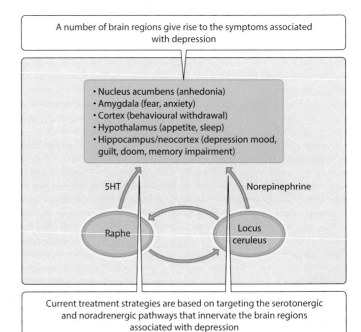

Fig. 3.36.1 Neuronal pathways of depression.

but they should not be given in combination with a MAO inhibitor.

Serotonin–norepinephrine reuptake inhibitors. **Venlafaxine** and **duloxetine** selectively inhibit the transport of serotonin and norepinephrine into their respective nerve terminals. Side-effects resemble those of SSRIs.

Norepinephrine reuptake inhibitor. **Reboxetine**, the only drug of this class, does not inhibit the transport of serotonin in serotonergic nerve terminals and can be used with SSRIs. Side-effects include dry mouth, constipation and insomnia.

Miscellaneous antidepressants

Mirtazapine. This agent blocks α_2-adrenoceptor auto-receptors present on cell bodies or presynaptic terminals and increases norepinephrine release from their neurons. As α-adrenoceptors are present on cell bodies (α_1-adrenoceptor) and terminal endings (α_2-adrenoceptor) of raphe serotonergic neurons, mirtazapine promotes serotonin release by augmenting noradrenergic activation of Raphe cell bodies and preventing terminal ending negative feedback. It also blocks excitatory $5HT_2$ and $5HT_3$ receptors on postsynaptic neurons, which may also account for its antidepressant activity. Side-effects are less than for SSRIs but it will cause drowsiness, sedation (H_1), appetite and weight gain (H_1, $5HT_{2C}$).

Atypical antidepressants. These include agents that block serotonin reuptake but are also $5HT_2$ receptor antagonists (**trazodone**, **nefazodone**). Side-effects include sedation, hypotension and reflex tachycardia. **Bupropion** inhibits norepinephrine and dopamine reuptake and is a $5HT_{1A}$ receptor agonist; its side-effects include dizziness, anxiety and seizures.

Mood stabilizers

Lithium carbonate is used in the treatment of bipolar affective disorders but also for the treatment of acute mania. It requires weeks to months to reduce manic episodes. At the biochemical level, lithium inhibits inositol monophosphatase, which disrupts the formation of the second messenger inositol 1,4,5-trisphosphate (IP_3), thereby decreasing postsynaptic sensitivity to neurotransmitters (e.g. serotonin). Other mechanisms of action have been proposed. Lithium has a narrow therapeutic window and major adverse effects include polyuria, hyper-thyroidism and weight gain. Toxicity manifests in the form of nausea, vomiting, diarrhoea, confusion, convulsions, coma and death. Anticonvulsants have also been used in the treatment of mania (**carbamazepine**, **valproate**).

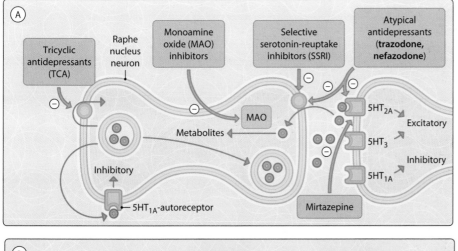

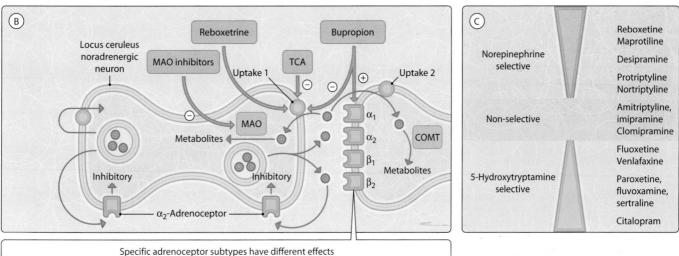

Fig. 3.36.2 Mechanisms of drug action. (A) Serotonergic antidepressants; (B) noradrenergic antidepressants; (C) selective effects on neurotransmitter reuptake.

37. Antipsychotic drugs and schizophrenia

Questions
- What is the characteristic feature of schizophrenia?
- What drugs are used in the treatment of schizophrenia?

Clinically, schizophrenia is characterized by hallucination and delusion (positive symptoms); apathy, unwillingness to socialize (negative symptoms); and cognitive deficits (lack of attention, decrease in memory). The finding that amphetamine could induce psychotic-like behaviour by stimulating dopamine release in the striatum and the beneficial effect of dopamine D_2 receptor antagonists in the treatment of this disease led to the proposal that schizophrenia results from an imbalance in dopaminergic neurotransmission (Fig. 3.37.1). However, it is appreciated that this disease is more complex and at a neurological level possibly related to a failure by dopaminergic, glutaminergic and GABAergic neurons to coordinate pyramidal firing patterns. Neuroimaging studies have revealed abnormal activity in the prefrontal cortex and increased (striatum) and reduced (cortex) dopaminergic activity. Therefore, the drugs used to treat this condition target dopamine and 5HT receptors, which helps to normalize glutaminergic and dopaminergic neurotransmission in schizophrenia.

Antipsychotic drugs are considered as two groups: the classical or typical drugs and the more recently developed atypical drugs (Fig. 3.37.1). The division is not clearly defined but relates to receptor profile, incidence of side-effects and efficacy in treating negative symptoms. Many antipyschotic drugs have:

- extrapyramidal side-effects (pertaining to brain areas concerned with motor coordination)
- sedative properties (antihistamine)
- prolactin-releasing action on pituitary (via D_2 receptors).

The atypical drugs are less prone to extrapyrimidal and endocrine side-effects probably because they have higher affinity for $5HT_{2A}$ receptors than for D_2 receptors.

Typical antipsychotic drugs

This diverse group of chemicals (phenothiazines, butyrophenones, thioxanthines) is effective in the treatment of the positive symptoms of schizophrenia and can have moderate activity on some aspects of negative symptoms and help to improve cognition. First-generation antipsychotic drugs produce an immediate blockade of D_2 receptors in all regions of the CNS and their clinical efficacy correlates with their affinity for D_2 and not D_1 receptors. Clinical benefit is evident some weeks after the

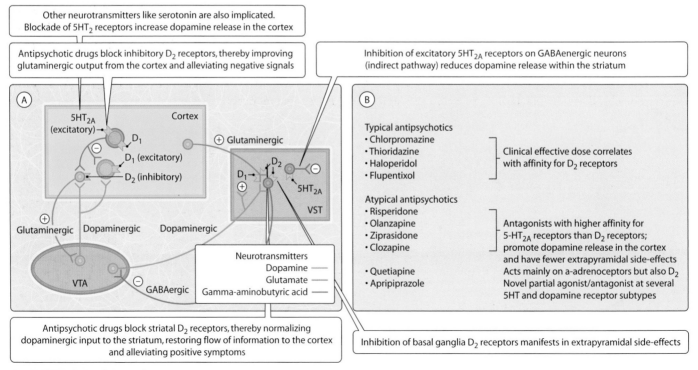

Fig. 3.37.1 Role of dopamine receptors.

commencement of drug treatment and suggests normalization of the complex interaction between the different neural pathways involved in cognition, memory, mood and behaviour. However, drugs such as **chlorpromazine fluphenazine, thiorazidine** (phenothiazine), **haloperidol** (butyrophenone), and **flupentixol** (thioxanthene) have diverse pharmacology and display affinity for different receptor types (e.g. α, H_1, M, $5HT_2$, D). This may account for their therapeutic beneficial activity (see atypical drugs below) and adverse actions.

Atypical antipsychotic drugs

Atypical antipsychotic drugs are D_2 receptor antagonists but their affinity for these receptors is lower than that of typical antipsychotic drugs and, consequently, they are less prone to cause the extrapyramidal side-effects characteristic of typical antipsychotic drugs. Like the typical antipsychotic drugs, these agents can ameliorate positive and negative symptoms and improve cognition.

> *Dibenzodiazepines.* **Clozapine** has low affinity for D_2 receptors but high affinity for $5HT_{2A}$ and D_4 receptors. Because dopamine content in the striatum is considerably greater than in the cortex, clozapine will be displaced from binding in the striatum and so extra-pyramidal side-effects will not occur. The beneficial action of clozapine in schizophrenia promoted the development of drugs with selectivity for dopamine (D_2) and serotonin ($5HT_2$) receptors. **Quetiapine, olanzepine, risperidone, zotepine** and **ziprasidone** have higher affinity for $5HT_2$ and D_2 receptors. In many cases, affinity is higher for $5HT_2$ than for D_2 receptors (risperidone, zotepine, ziprasidone) or for α-adrenoceptors (quetiapine, risperidone). These agents preferentially increase dopamine neurotransmission in the mesocortical pathway relative to the mesolimbic pathway (presumably through weak D_2 antagonism in striatum).

> *Partial agonists.* Recently approved for the treatment of schizophrenia, **aripiprazole** has higher affinity for D_2 and D_3 receptors than many atypical antipsychotic drugs but also documents affinity for $5HT_{1A,2A,7}$ receptors. More importantly, unlike many atypical antipsychotic drugs, aripiprazole can behave as a partial agonist, agonist and antagonist at these receptors sites. Whatever the precise mechanism for this behaviour, aripiprazole reduces dopaminergic neurotransmission in the striatum while increasing neurotransmission in the cortex.

> *D_2 and D_3 receptor antagonists.* A variety of substituted benzamides including and **sulpiride** and **amisulpride** are highly specific inhibitors of D_2 and D_3 receptors and have no activity on $5HT_{2A}$ receptors.

Side-effects of antipsychotic drugs

The major adverse action attributed to typical but not atypical antipsychotic drugs is the extrapyramidal side-effects, which give rise to a Parkinson-like disorder with uncoordinated motor activity (e.g. tremor, bradykinesia, dystonia and akathisia) through D_2 receptor antagonism in the nigrostriatal pathway. Some individuals can also develop severe neuroleptic malignant syndrome with typical antipsychotic drugs, resulting in body temperatures in excess of 40°C; this can be treated with a dopamine agonist, **bromocriptine**. Typical antipsychotic drugs can also increase the release of prolactin from the anterior pituitary by blocking inhibitory postsynaptic D_2 receptors. The high serum concentrations of prolactin can lead to galactorrhoea, amenorrhoea and infertility. Both typical and atypical antipsychotic drugs demonstrate a number of side-effects owing to their non-selectivity, including sedation (H_1), dry mouth (muscarinic), postural hypotension (α_1), weight gain and associated metabolic side-effects (H_1, α_1, $5HT_{2C}$). Only clozapine causes agranulocytosis.

38. Antiseizure agents and epilepsy

Questions
- What is the characteristic feature of epilepsy?
- What drugs are used in the treatment of epilepsy?

Epilepsy is characterized by seizures broadly classified as generalized or partial (localized) syndromes (Fig. 3.38.1). The simultaneous activation of both hemispheres characterize generalized epilepsy, which is manifested as a convulsive seizure with periods of muscle rigidity (tonic) followed by jerking of the body (clonic), commonly referred to as a tonic–clonic (or grand mal) seizure. In childhood absence epilepsy, subjects frequently lose consciousness for brief moments without recollection of the event and are non-convulsive. The molecular basis of the generalized syndromes is not fully understood, although it may involve mutations in various ion channels (sodium, $GABA_A$) and an abnormality in the thalamic relay sensory unit (thalamo-cortical pathway) resulting in neuronal hyperexcitability. Partial

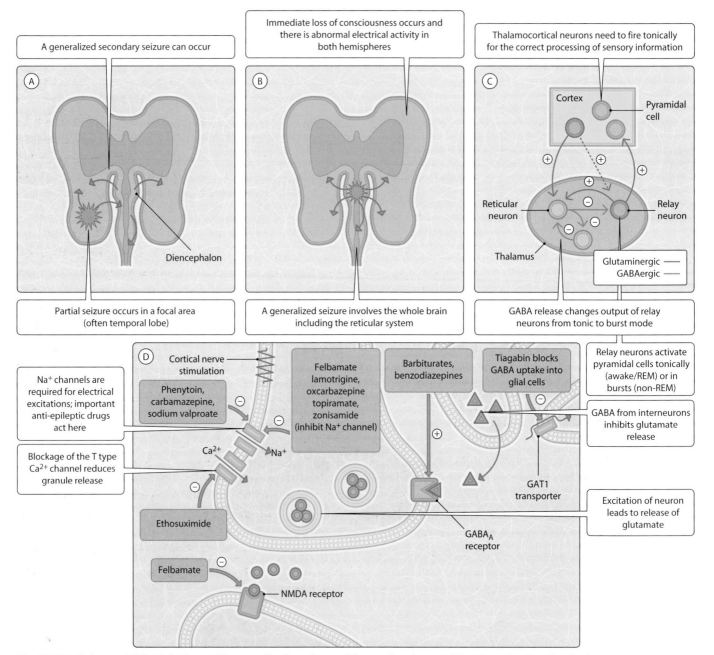

Fig. 3.38.1 Seizures. (A) Partial seizure; (B) generalized syndrome; (C) neural pathways; (D) action of anti-epileptic drugs.

syndromes are most common in adults, with the seizure beginning in a particular location (e.g. temporal lobe as a result of a stroke) and spreading throughout the brain. Temporal lobe seizures are characterized by hallucination, confusion and loss of awareness. If the focus is localized in the motor cortex, then tonic–clonic seizures can result.

Drug treatment

The major aim of treatment is to reduce neuronal hyper-excitability and this is achieved by targeting GABA$_A$, sodium and calcium channels (Fig. 3.38.1D).

Established anti-epileptic agents

Phenytoin. Phenytoin preferentially binds to the inactivated state of the sodium channels in a use-dependent manner and delays their recovery from this inactivated state. This reduces the frequency of channel opening and neuronal excitability. It is given orally for the treatment of generalized and partial epilepsy with the exception of absence seizure. Phenytoin induces hepatic cytochrome P450 activity and, therefore, increases the metabolism of other drugs including anticoagulants, contraceptives, dexamethasone and pethidine. Adverse actions include sedation and confusion (acute toxicity), ataxia, hyperactivity, rash, hepatitis and megaloblastic anaemia.

Carbamazepine. Structurally related to tricyclic anti-depressants, carbamazepine like phenytoin blocks sodium channels. It is administered orally for most epilepsy with the exception of absence seizure. Carbamazepine also induces cytochrome P450 activity in the liver and, therefore, affects the metabolism of both itself and other drugs. Side-effects include ataxia, vertigo and sedation.

Sodium valproate. This has a similar mechanism of action to phenytoin. Valproate also elevates GABA levels throughout the brain; it is a weak inhibitor of GABA transaminase and, therefore, inhibits the degradation of GABA. Valproate has a better safety profile than traditionally used agents but is hepatotoxic and should not be given to individuals with liver dysfunction. Major side-effects include gastrointestinal disturbances. **Vigabatrine** is a newer anti-epileptic drug that is an irreversible inhibitor of GABA transaminase.

Barbiturates. Barbiturates (e.g. **phenobarbital**) have sedative, anaesthetic and anticonvulsant activity, although their use in epilepsy is limited because better tolerated drugs have been developed. Phenobarbital binds to an allosteric site on the GABA$_A$ chloride channel, resulting in channel opening and membrane hyperpolarization. It is usually administered orally for most forms of epilepsy apart from absence epilepsy. It is administered i.v. in emergency (status epilepticus). Phenobarbital is a strong inducer of cytochrome P450, is likely to produce CNS depression and can be fatal with overdose; consequently, it is not suitable for use in children, the elderly or those with respiratory depression.

Benzodiazepines. Benzodiazepines (**diazepam**, **clonazepam** and **lorazepam**) bind to the α-subunit of the GABA$_A$ chloride channels and increase the probability of channel opening in response to GABA; they differ from barbiturates, which can open the GABA$_A$ chloride channel directly. These drugs are useful in absence seizures and are administered i.v. in emergency for status epilepticus (diazepam). A major side-effect is sedation, and tolerance can develop with prolonged usage.

Ethosuximide. This drug inhibits voltage-dependent T-type calcium channels, which are predominantly found in the thalamocortical relay neurons, and, therefore, is used in the treatment of absence seizures. The activation of T-type (low-threshold) channels is responsible for the generation of the 3 Hz spike and wave discharge seen in absence seizure. It is well tolerated and adverse effects include gastrointestinal upset, drowsiness and skin rashes.

New anti-epileptic agents

A number of agents are also available for use in the treatment of epilepsy. They demonstrate non-selective pharmacology and are approved for use in partial seizures, generalized seizure (**felbamate, lamotrigine, topiramate**) and in absence seizure (**zonisamide**) as adjuncts with other therapies. A number of the newer anti-epileptic drugs are used as monotherapy (felbamate, lamotrigine, **oxcarbazepine**). The main advantage of these drugs over traditional anti-epileptic agents is their lack of induction of cytochrome P450, so not affecting the metabolism of other drugs; therefore, they are better tolerated. Adverse affects associated with these agents include aplastic anaemia, hepatoxicity and gastrointestinal disturbances (felbamate, which may limit its use); dizziness, fatigue and somnolence (**gabapetin**, topiramate, **levetiracetam**, oxcarbazepine); rash (lamotrigine, which is exacerbated if used in conjunction with valproate as this anticonvulsant slows the metabolism of lamotrigine); and hyponatraemia (oxcarbazepine). Zonisamide is contradicted in sulphonamide allergy as it is a sulphonamide derivative.

39. General anaesthetics

Questions
- What is general anaesthesia?
- What drugs are used to produce the various stages of general anaesthesia?

General anaesthesia is the loss of awareness of sensory inputs resulting in analgesia, unconsciousness (sedation and hypnosis), amnesia and immobilization. The loss of consciousness and amnesia is a consequence of suppression of neuronal excitability in various brain regions (e.g. midbrain reticular formation, thalamus) while loss of mobility results from depression of spinal neurons. Neuronal conduction is not sensitive to general anaesthetic agents, and the peripheral axons of motor neurons distal to the spinal cord do not contribute to immobility nor do these drugs directly inhibit neuromuscular transmission. The higher centres of the brain are more susceptible to general anaesthetics and as a consequence sedation, hypnosis and amnesia can be achieved at much lower concentrations than that required to prevent movement in response to a surgical incision and the autonomic response to pain. General anaesthesia is achieved with a combination of i.v. and inhalational drugs. Other agents may also be administered as premedication (Fig. 3.39.1).

Volatile anaesthetics
Volatile general anaesthetics include the halogenated hydro-carbons (**halothane**), halogenated ethers (**sevoflurane, desflurane, enflurane, isofluorane**) and non-carbon-based gases (**nitrous oxide**). While the potency of inhalational anaesthetics correlates with lipid solubility (Meyer–Overton rule, Fig. 3.39.2),

exceptions to this rule shifted attention from membrane lipids to proteins, and it is now recognized that binding to proteins in neuronal membranes alters their gating kinetics. Volatile anaesthetics enhance the activity of $GABA_A$ and glycine receptors, thereby facilitating hyperpolarization and reducing neuronal excitability. Volatile anaesthetics can also inhibit the function of receptors (e.g. NMDA, nicotinic) that increase postsynaptic channel activity (Fig. 3.39.3).

Nitrous oxide. Nitrous oxide (laughing gas) is a non-flammable volatile general anaesthetic with low blood solubility and, hence, the rate of induction and recovery from anaesthesia is rapid. It is often used in combination with other anaesthetics as it cannot produce surgical anaesthesia nor does it induce skeletal muscle relaxation when administered alone because of its lack of potency. Since it is not metabolized by the liver and is eliminated by the lung, it is free from side-effects and is, therefore, used as an adjunct. This allows the use of lower concentrations of other inhalational anaesthetics, thereby reducing their potential for adverse effects. Nitrous oxide produces little cardiovascular or respiratory depression when used alone. Prolonged exposure impairs methionine synthase, a vitamin B_{12}-dependent enzyme, and so will interfere with DNA synthesis in rapidly proliferating cells in the bone marrow (leukocytes, red blood cells).

Halothane. Halothane is a non-flammable halogenated ether that is highly soluble in blood and, therefore, has slower induction and recovery phases compared with nitrous oxide. It is used in combination with analgesics and muscle

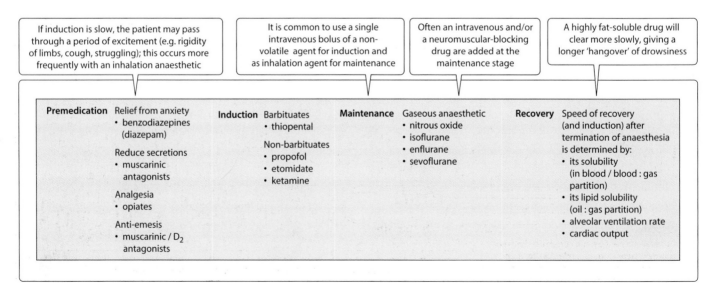

Fig. 3.39.1 Sequence of general anaesthesia.

relaxants as it does not produce analgesia and has variable action on muscle relaxation. Halothane accumulates within body fat, which further delays recovery. It is metabolized within the liver and the active metabolites can cause hepatic necrosis (halothane hepatitis) in susceptible individuals. Halothane produces a fall in blood pressure through a reduction in cardiac output and respiratory depression necessitates the use of mechanical ventilation to compensate for the rise in arterial levels of carbon dioxide. The use of halothane has declined in favour of more potent and better tolerated gaseous anaesthetics.

Enflurane. Enflurane has a lower solubility in blood than halothane and so has a quicker induction and recovery rate; it also produces muscle relaxation. It is much less hepatotoxic than halothane as it is metabolized to a lesser degree (2–10%). Like halothane, enflurane also produces cardiac and respiratory depression.

Isoflurane. An isomer of enflurane but with a lower blood: gas solubility coefficient, iosflurane has considerably lower hepatoxicity as only 0.2% is metabolized by the liver. It also produces a decrease in systemic blood pressure through vasodilatation in skin and skeletal muscle but does not reduce cardiac output.

Sevoflurane. As sevoflurane has low solubility in blood compared with isoflurane, it provides rapid induction and recovery from anaesthesia. It also undergoes metabolism by the liver (3%) but, despite this, the reports of hepatic injury are rare. Compared with the other inhaled anaesthetics, sevoflurane produces less cardiopulmonary depression.

Intravenous anaesthetics

Intravenous general anaesthetics include the barbiturate **thiopental** and non-barbiturates **propofol**, **etomidate** (GABA receptor) and **ketamine**.

Propofol. This is the most common anaesthetic agent for i.v. use and causes rapid induction of anaesthesia. It is also associated with rapid recovery from anaesthesia without nausea or hangover effect and is rapidly metabolized by the liver. In rare cases, some individuals demonstrate allergic response on a subsequent exposure. Anaesthesia is maintained with continuous infusion and used in combination with opiates and other inhalational anaesthetics.

Etomidate. Like propofol, etomidate causes rapid induction from anaesthesia without nausea and hangover. It also can cause an allergic reaction in susceptible individuals. Pain upon injection and extraneous muscle movement are unwanted side-effects.

Ketamine. What is referred to as disassociated anaesthesia is produced by ketamine, where patients may remain conscious but are insensitive to pain; it also produces amnesia and paralysis of movement. It does not cause muscle relaxation and its use is limited by cardiovascular stimulant actions and high incidence of hallucination during recovery from anaesthesia.

Thiopental. Thiopental causes rapid induction (less than 30 s) and recovery from anaesthesia. It does produce respiratory depression and has transient effects on blood pressure. Inadvertent intra-arterial injection with high concentrations of thiopental will cause spasm.

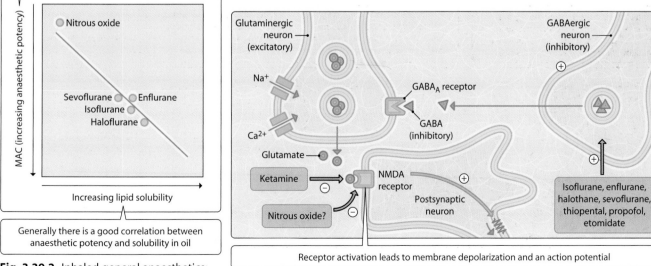

Fig. 3.39.2 Inhaled general anaesthetics: the Meyer–Overton rule.

Fig. 3.39.3 Molecular targets of general anaesthetics.

40. Migraine

Questions
- What is a migraine?
- What is the pharmacological treatment of migraine?

Migraine is characterized by pulsating severe headache of long duration (4–72 h) and is often accompanied by nausea and sensitivity to light, sound or movement (common migraine). At least 20% of patients suffer from migraine with aura (classic migraine) and this is preceded by neurological symptoms (e.g. visual). These features distinguish migraine from tension-type headache, the most common form of primary headache. The mechanisms underlying a migraine are thought to arise as a combination of cranial vessel constriction (aura) and dilatation (pain, headache), although it is clear that cerebral blood flow is altered during a migraine attack. During an attack, there is a brief wave of intense cortical stimulation followed by marked depression of cortical activity, which lasts for up to an hour and spreads across the surface of the brain. Reduced blood flow (oligaemia) develops in this area of cortical depression, which gives rise to headache. There is also evidence that the spreading cortical depression may sensitize trigeminovascular afferent neurons, which would facilitate cranial vessel dilatation and transmission of impulses to higher centres and the expression of pain and headache (Fig. 3.40.1A).

Management of acute attacks

NSAIDs. NSAIDs (e.g. ibuprofen can be useful in the treatment of headache associated with migraine and are administered when headache is first recognized (Fig. 3.40.1C). The role of prostaglandins in sensitization of nociceptive afferent neurons is the basis for their beneficial mechanism of action. The utility of this treatment varies between patients and severity of migraine.

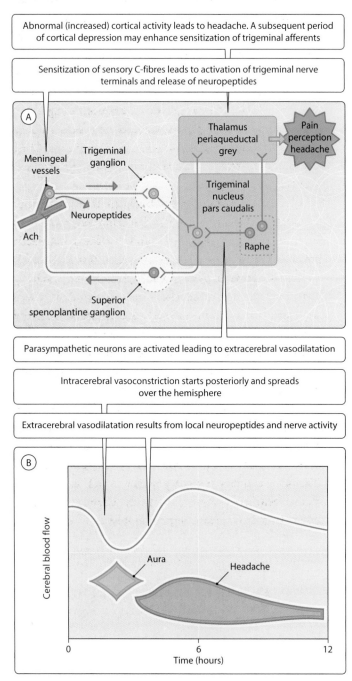

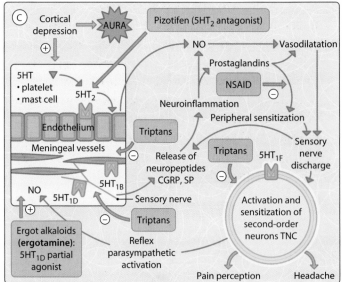

Fig. 3.40.1 Migraine. (A) Proposed mechanism; (B) cerebral blood flow; (C) postulated pathogenesis and drugs acting in acute attacks.

Ergot derivatives.   **Ergotamine** offers a low cost approach to the treatment of acute attacks of migraine. It has a complex pharmacology and is a partial agonist at α_1-adrenoceptor and $5HT_{1D}$ receptors, thereby promote meningeal vasoconstriction. Ergotamine is susceptible to first pass metabolism and is more likely to induce nausea (D_2 agonism in area postrema) following oral administration, which can be minimized by using it as a rectal suppository. Ergotamine is contraindicated in pregnant women and in patients with peripheral vascular disease, coronary heart disease, hypertension and impaired hepatic or renal function.

Triptans.   Unlike the ergot derivatives, the triptans (e.g. **sumatriptan**, **naratriptan**, **zolmitriptan**) have a selective pharmacology for serotonin receptors. Triptans are selective agonists for $5HT_{1B,1D}$ receptors but they are also selective for $5HT_{1F}$ receptors and therapeutic action at this receptor should not be ruled out. Activation of $5HT$ receptors results in vasoconstriction ($5HT_{1B}$), inhibition of neuropeptide release from sensory neurons ($5HT_{1D}$) and inhibition of second-order neurons in the brainstem ($5HT_{1F}$). These drugs are administered orally and are metabolized in the liver, with peak plasma concentration achieved 1–4 h after ingestion. The most frequent side-effect includes tingling and sensations of warmth in the upper body. Triptans can cause vasoconstriction of the coronary arteries, giving rise to chest pains resembling those of angina pectoris. In rare cases, treatment with these drugs is associated with myocardial infarction. They are, therefore, contraindicated in ischaemic heart disease, uncontrolled hypertension and cerebrovascular disease.

Other agents.   The clinical utility of NSAIDs is evident in pain of mild severity, although stronger non-narcotic formulations may be of use in the treatment of migraine. A combination of **paracetamol** (acetaminophen) or **aspirin** with a mild vasoconstrictor (**isometheptene**) or sedative (**butalbital**; short-acting barbiturate) can be used. There are concerns with the use of a vasoconstrictor (contraindicated in glaucoma, hypertension and heart disease) and butalbital (potentially addictive). Nausea is a characteristic feature of migraine and can be treated with anti-emetic agents (e.g. **metoclopramide**).

Prophylactic management

In some individuals, migraine may be triggered by certain foods and beverages, including chocolate, cheese, red wine, nuts, preserved meats and fish. Regular sleep can also reduce the risk of migraine attack. Too little or too much sleep can increase the risk of migraine and may be related to alterations in brain serotonin levels. A number of pharmacological agents can be used prophylactically to minimize the incidence of migraine and should be used when a patient has three or more attacks a month or when the attacks are severe enough and the accompanying symptoms (nausea, photophobia) become disabling.

Beta-blockers.   There is convincing evidence supporting the prophylactic use of beta-blockers for the prevention of migraine. **Propranolol** and **timolol** are effective while beta-blockers with intrinsic sympathomimetic activity (partial agonists, e.g. **alprenolol**, **oxprenolol** and **pindolol**) are without effect. The exact site of action has not been determined and there is experimental evidence to suggest an action on β_1-adrenoceptors in the thalamus. Beta-blockers are contraindicated in asthma and congestive heart failure; common side-effects include hypotension, lethargy and gastrointestinal upset.

Anticonvulsants.   **Divalproex sodium** (1:1 ratio of sodium valproate and valproic acid) and **sodium valproate** have been shown to be of clinical utility in the prophylactic treatment of migraine. The exact mechanism of action is unclear but these drugs may reduce the cortical excitability that precedes the headache seen in migraine. These anticonvulsants enhance GABAergic inhibitory activity (inhibit GABA transaminase) and inhibit sodium and calcium channels, which would serve to reduce neuronal excitability. Other anticonvulsants including topiramate and vigabatrin may be of some clinical utility.

Antidepressants.   **Amitriptyline** and **nortriptyline** are tricyclic antidepressants that have proved to be efficacious in migraine. The mechanism of action is not completely understood and is independent of antidepressant action. The other antidepressants types have little if any demonstrable beneficial action. Side-effects include drowsiness, weight gain and anticholinergic symptoms.

41. Treatment of pain

Questions
- What are the pathways involved in the perception of pain?
- What drugs are used to treat pain?

The perception of pain is a normal defence mechanism in order to avoid further harm. Pain arising under pathological situations (e.g. neuropathic pain) can be seriously debilitating and is characterized by an increase in perception of innocuous (allodynia) or noxious (hyperalgesia) stimuli. Peripheral sensory nerve endings (C, Aδ) present in the skin and viscera respond to mechanical, chemical or thermal stimuli. The activation of these neurons results in the release of neuropeptides and glutamate from their terminal endings in the vicinity of dorsal horn neurons (laminae I, II, IV–VI). The release of neuropeptides and glutamate from the spinal terminals of these afferent nerves activates dorsal horn neurons that, in turn, relay neurotransmission centrally where pain is perceived (Fig. 3.41.1). Acute or chronic pain is a consequence of an increase in pain neurotransmission. Endogenous opioids regulate pain transmission by (a) activating supraspinal regions (e.g. thalamus) and thereby reducing pain perception; (b) activating the periaqueductal grey and rostroventrial medulla (VRM) and thereby increasing the inhibitory activity of the descending pathway; (c) directly inhibiting dorsal horn neurons by enkephalin-releasing interneurons; and (d) inhibiting neuropeptide and glutamate release from peripheral sensory nerves synapsing with dorsal horn neurons. Endogenous opioids regulate pain transmission by activating G-protein-coupled receptors present on spinal and supraspinal nerves. There are three receptor subtypes, μ (mu), κ (kappa) and δ (delta), which are activated by endogenous opioids (e.g. met-enkephalin, β-endorphin). The μ receptor subtypes mediate most of the analgesic actions of opioids.

Opioids

A variety of synthetic opioid analogues based on the structure of the naturally occurring opioid morphine have clinical efficacy in the treatment and management of pain (Fig. 3.41.1C). These agonists are relatively selective for and bind reversibly to opioid μ receptors, which couple to potassium channels and result in membrane hyperpolarization, reduced neuronal excitability and inhibition of neurotransmitter release (e.g. neuropeptide, glutamate). In contrast, local anaesthetics and NSAIDs (but not opioids) reduce pain by inhibiting nerve conduction and sensitization of peripheral nerve endings by prostaglandins, respectively. There are a number of different structural classes of opioid receptor agonist (see below). While opioids are generally used for analgesia, there are examples of opioids used for other indications (e.g. constipation and cough). Examples of partial μ-opioid agonists and antagonists include **buprenorphine** and **naloxone**, respectively.

Morphine and morphine-related opioids. These are widely used to relieve moderate-to-severe pain and frequently used to relieve chronic pain in patients with cancer, terminally ill patients and in the management of postoperative pain (e.g. **morphine**, **heroin**, **codeine**, **hydrocodone**, **oxycodone**). In mild-to-moderate pain, codeine is frequently used together with an NSAID (e.g. aspirin or paracetamol).

Pethidine -like opioids. Pethidine (meperidine) is also widely used in the treatment of moderate-to-severe pain while the pethidine-like agent **loperamide** is used only as an anti-diarrhoeal agent (it slows gastrointestinal transit and reduces secretions, making it useful for the treatment of diarrhoea). Loperamide has low solubility, undergoes enterohepatic recycling and has considerably reduced ability to cross the blood–brain barrier; this accounts for its lack of analgesic properties and low substance abuse potential.

Fentanyl, alfentanil and sufentanil. Fentanyl and its derivatives alfentanil and sufentanil are considerably more potent than morphine and provide rapid analgesia following i.v. administration. These agents are, therefore, useful in premedication for surgical procedures.

Methodone-related opioids. Methodone is structurally unrelated to morphine and is an analgesic with prolonged duration of action, making it very useful in reducing the physical symptoms in drug addicts who are being treated for their drug dependency.

Side-effects

The presence of opioid receptors within the CNS accounts for the side-effects of these drugs, including sedation, reduced anxiety and, in some cases, euphoria and respiratory depression. Opiates may also induce hypotension through action on the medulla or through peripheral vasodilatation caused by mast cell degranulation and release of histamine (morphine). The signs of opiate overdose include miosis, respiratory depression and coma. Tolerance to chronic opiate administration can develop for analgesia, respiratory depression and emesis, but not for constipation or miosis. This may be related to alterations in the number of opioid receptors. Psychological (nervousness, sweating and craving) and physical (cramps, pupil dilatation, diarrhoea, depression) dependence manifests after withdrawal

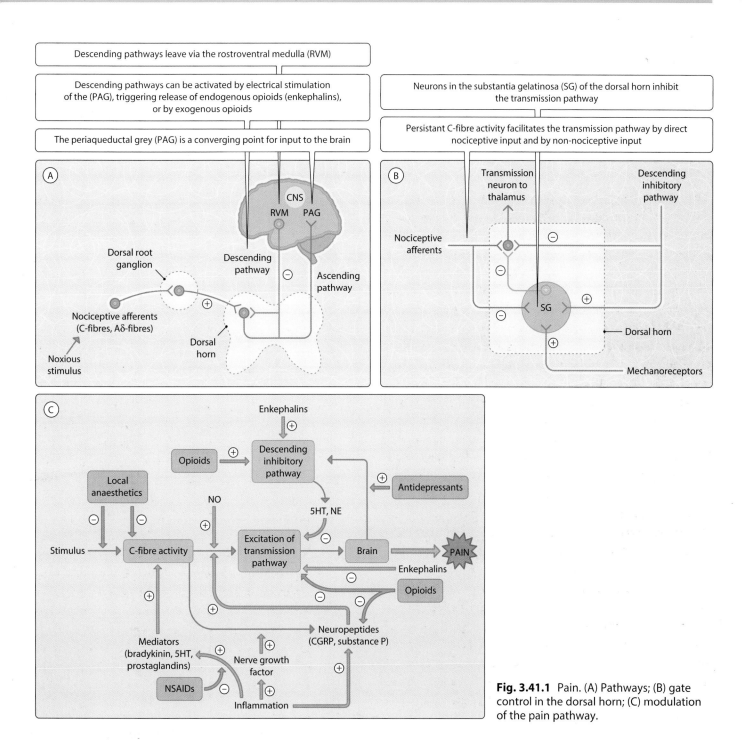

Fig. 3.41.1 Pain. (A) Pathways; (B) gate control in the dorsal horn; (C) modulation of the pain pathway.

of opioids following chronic use (or following substance abuse). Methadone is often used in these circumstances as the drug has a long half-life, thereby reducing the intensity of these symptoms.

Metabolism

In general, opioids are readily absorbed across the gastrointestinal tract and following parenteral administration. Morphine undergoes glucuronidation in the liver to morphine 6-glucuronide, which has considerably greater potency than morphine. However, this metabolite crosses the blood–brain barrier less readily. Codeine is also subject to first pass metabolism and a small fraction is demethylated in the liver to

morphine, which accounts for the analgesic actions of this agent. Highly potent opioids like fentanyl, alfentanil and sufentanil have rapid onset of action (rapid entry into CNS) but are extensively bound to plasma protein and redistribute to peripheral tissue, hence their shorter durations of action.

Other agents used in the management of pain

There are many drug classes that are used in the management of pain syndromes, including NSAIDs, tricyclic antidepressants, anticonvulsants and local anaesthetics (Fig. 3.41.1C). More information concerning the pharmacology of these drug classes is given in the relevant chapters.

42. Substances of abuse

Questions

- What are the pathways involved in drug addiction?
- What substances cause drug addiction and how are they treated?

A number of substances repeatedly taken either legally (nicotine, alcohol) or illegally (amphetamine, cocaine, heroin) can give rise to substance dependence. Substances of abuse increase the mesocortical and mesolimbic dopaminergic pathways associated with salience and reward for natural drives (e.g. food, water and sex) that originate in the ventral tegmental area (VTA) and project to the prefrontal cortex and limbic system. Neuroadaptive changes promote craving, compulsion for drug taking, conditioned response (i.e. cues) linked to craving (e.g. desire to smoke in a social setting), tolerance and withdrawal symptoms (Fig. 3.42.1).

Opiates

Opioids (heroin, morphine) disinhibit dopaminergic activity in the VTA by stimulating opioid μ receptors on GABAergic interneurons, increasing dopamine levels within nucleus accumbens and VTA. They produce euphoria, sedation and tranquillity when administered acutely. Chronic uncontrolled use gives rise to craving (psychological dependence), tolerance and withdrawal symptoms, which include irritability, aggression, sweating, restlessness, pupil dilatation and piloerection (giving rise to the euphemism 'cold turkey'). In overdose, they cause lethal respiratory depression. **Methadone** is a weak agonist of the opioid μ receptor and is used to treat heroin addiction as it reduces the severity and manifestation of withdrawal symptoms and craving. Extended exposure to methadone produces cross-tolerance (desensitization) and this, in a sense, antagonizes the pharmacological action of heroin. Furthermore, its longer plasma half-life also accounts for a reduction of the symptoms associated with withdrawal. **Buprenorphine** is a partial opioid μ receptor agonist that has a slower onset of action and longer duration of action than heroin. Like methadone, it provides cross-tolerance to the actions of heroin and has the added advantage that unintentional overdose is avoided. **Naltrexone** is a opioid μ receptor antagonist that directly blocks the actions of opiates. This distinct mechanism of action makes the drug

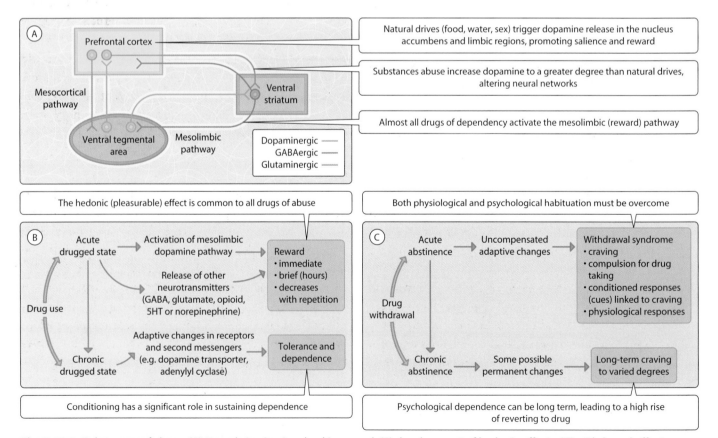

Fig. 3.42.1 Substances of abuse. (A) Neural circuitry involved in reward; (B) development of hedonic effects; (C) withdrawal effects.

useful in the treatment of heroin addiction, particularly when accompanied with behavioural treatment.

CNS stimulants

Amphetamines.   Amphetamines act by inhibiting reuptake of dopamine and norepinephrine into nerve terminals, inhibiting monoamine oxidase and promoting release of dopamine and norepinephrine. Acute administration of the psychostimulant amphetamine produces feelings of euphoria, arousal, increased alertness, concentration and motor activity. Amphetamine causes strong psychological dependence, and withdrawal syndromes include depression and sleep disturbance. Blood pressure is increased via action on the peripheral sympathetic nervous system. Long-term use gives rise to irritability, aggression, stereotypical behaviour and paranoid-like psychosis.

Cocaine.   Cocaine increases dopamine levels by inhibiting reuptake of dopamine, norepinephrine and serotonin into nerve terminals. The elevation of these neurotransmitters in synaptic sites is implicated in substance dependence. Animal studies implicate a role for serotonin and norepinephrine. The behavioural effects are similar to those described for amphetamine; cocaine causes strong psychological dependence, and mild withdrawal syndromes includes depression and sleep disturbance.

'Ecstasy' (methylenedioxymethamphetamine; MDMA).   This designer drug derived from amphetamine produces euphoria and increases empathy. Acute toxicity results in cerebral haemorrhage, hyperthermia, heat stroke, panic and psychosis. MDMA inhibits serotonin reuptake.

CNS depressants

Ethanol.   Ethanol promotes $GABA_A$ receptor inhibitory activity and acts as an NMDA receptor antagonist on glutaminergic neurons, increasing dopaminergic activity in the VTA. At low doses, its action is stimulatory via suppression of central inhibitory systems. As the concentration of ethanol increases, CNS depression is characterized by sedation, motor incoordination and impaired psychomotor performance. Withdrawal symptoms can range from mild (anxiety, agitation, tremor, sweating and nausea) to severe (seizures and delirium tremens). Approved pharmacological treatments for alcoholism include **acamprosate**, which is thought to act as an NMDA receptor antagonist, reducing ethanol signalling. The receptor antagonist

naltrexone is effective in the treatment of alcoholism and may block endogenous opioid-dependent pathways. The efficacy of this treatment is increased when accompanied by behavioural treatment.

Benzodiazepines.   Benzodiazepines are discussed in Ch. 35. They are used in anxiety and as sedatives, anticonvulsants and premedication for surgery. Chronic use leads to tolerance, and withdrawal symptoms include rebound anxiety, insomnia, depression and nausea.

Hallucinogens

Hallucinogens or psychotomimetic drugs include lysergic acid diethylamide (LSD), mescaline and phencyclidine. They alter perception, thought and mood by provoking psychomotor stimulation or depression. LSD is a partial agonist at $5HT_{2A}$ receptors and alters the firing pattern of serotonergic neurons. It alters perceptions particularly those associated with sight and sound and produces hallucination, which can, in susceptible individuals, precipitate schizophrenia. LSD is not associated with tolerance, dependence or withdrawal symptoms.

Cannabinoids

The active constituent of marijuana, Δ^9-tetrahydrocannabinol (THC), has affinity for CB_1 receptors on GABAergic and glutaminergic neurons to the VTA, increasing dopaminergic firing and dopamine release. Marijuana produces feelings of well-being and relaxation and impairs cognitive function; in overdose it can cause panic attacks. Chronic use is associated with impaired memory function, loss of energy and drive. Tolerance develops to a minor extent and it is not overtly addictive. Withdrawal symptoms are only seen in heavy users, characterized by restlessness, irritability and insomnia.

Nicotine

Nicotine stimulates nicotinic receptors on VTA dopaminergic neurons, promoting dopamine release in the limbic system. This increases alertness, reduces irritability and relaxes skeletal smooth muscle (inhibits spinal reflexes). Tolerance develops to the peripheral and central actions of nicotine. Nicotine consumption leads to craving and withdrawal symptoms that include irritability, anxiety and increased appetite. Pharmacological treatment for addiction includes **bupropion**, which inhibits serotonin and norepinephrine transport into nerve terminals and is moderately effective.

43. Chemotherapy: antibiotics targeting cell wall and nucleic acid synthesis

Questions
- What are the targets for antibiotics?
- What problems occur with the β-lactam antibiotics?

The term chemotherapy was initially used to describe the use of synthetic chemicals to destroy infective agents, but it has been broadened to include antibiotics (agents produced by microorganisms to inhibit the action of other microorganisms) and their synthetic derivatives and still further to cover the use of chemicals to kill cancer cells. Antibiotics kill bacteria (bacteriocidal) or inhibit growth (bacteriostatic) and allow the body's natural immune system to eliminate the invading organism. Antibacterial agents target essential pathways necessary for bacterial growth and survival:

- the cell wall (e.g. penicillin)
- cell membrane permeability (e.g. amphotericin)
- nucleic acids (e.g. DNA unwinding (fluoroquinines))
- synthesis of building blocks (sulphonamides)
- protein synthesis (e.g. tetracyclines; Ch. 44).

Agents affecting cell wall

The cell membranes of Gram-negative and Gram-positive bacteria are composed of layers of peptidoglycans cross-linked with short amino acid chains; transpeptidase catalyses this cross-linking (Fig. 3.43.1). The β-lactam antibiotics (e.g. penicillins, cephalosporins, monobactams and carbapenems (Fig. 3.43.1C) covalently bind to the active site of this enzyme via the β-lactam ring moiety and reduce its catalytic activity. The resulting disruption of the cell wall results in cell swelling, rupture and bacteriocidal activity through the inability to maintain an osmotic gradient across the membrane. This class of antibiotic is susceptible to enzymatic cleavage by β-lactamases, which are produced by some bacteria and protects them from this type of bacteriocidal activity, thus conferring resistance.

Benzylpenicillin (penicillin G) is a broad-spectrum antibiotic and is often the first choice of therapy, but it suffers from poor oral bioavailability, so must be injected, and is susceptible to bacterial β-lactamases. Semisynthetic penicillins have been produced commercially that have oral bioavailability plus broad (**amoxicillin**) and extended (**ticarcillin**) spectra of activities and greater resistance to β-lactamases (**flucloxacillin**). An

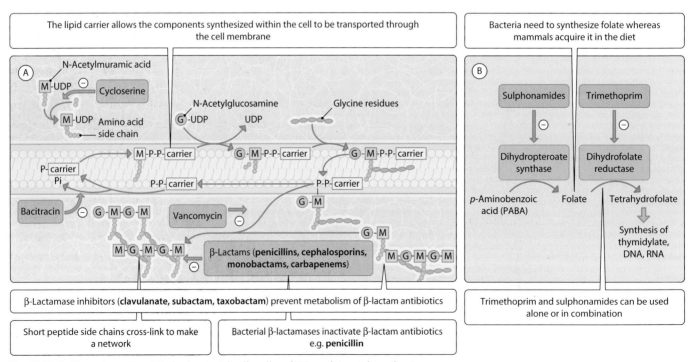

Fig. 3.43.1 Drugs targeting (A) the bacterial cell wall and (B) nucleic acid synthesis.

alternative approach is to combine the penicillin with a β-lactamase inhibitor (see below) to improve antimicrobial activity. The plasma half-life of penicillin can be improved with **probenecid**, which inhibits its renal excretion.

Other β-lactams, including carbapenems (imipenem) and monobactams (aztreonam), have been developed in an attempt to avoid or minimize metabolism by β-lactamase. Carbapenems have broad spectrum of activity against Gram-positive and Gram-negative bacteria, while the monobactams are only effective against aerobic Gram-negative bacteria and are insensitive to β-lactamases. Major adverse reactions to β-lactams include hypersensitivity reactions (e.g. rash), anaphylaxis (rare) and gastrointestinal disturbance owing to inhibition of gastrointestinal flora.

Vancomycin (glycoprotein) inhibits cell wall synthesis but at an earlier stage of the formation of the peptidoglycan layer than β-lactams (Fig. 3.43.1A). As a consequence, resistance is rare, although vancomycin-resistant *Staphylococcus aureus* has been reported. Vancomycin interferes with the elongation of peptidoglycan chains by covalently binding to the terminal endings of pentapeptide residues, which undergo the cross-linking reaction by transpeptidase. It is only active against Gram-positive bacteria as it is too large to access across cell walls of Gram-negative bacteria. This agent has the advantage of not being susceptible to β-lactamases and, therefore, of use in β-lactam-resistant bacterial strains (e.g. methicillin-resistant *S. aureus* (MSRA) and penicillin-resistant pneumococci). It has poor oral bioavailability and is administered i.v. (orally for intestinal infection). Side-effects include fever, rash and nephrotoxicity at high plasma levels.

A number of agents that contain a β-lactam ring covalently bind to and inactivate β-lactamases. They are not bactericidal but prevent the metabolism of β-lactam antibiotics and are, therefore, used in combination therapy (Fig. 3.43.1A).

Agents affecting nucleic acid synthesis

The enzyme topoisomerase II (DNA gyrase) is necessary for DNA replication. All bacterial DNA are circular molecules and this enzyme adjusts DNA topographically by supercoiling it into tight stable negative coils. It also breaks and reseals DNA strands to relieve tension as the DNA molecule replicates. Fluoroquinolones are selective inhibitors of bacterial but not mammalian topoisomerase and are bacteriocidal with broad-spectrum antimicrobial activity. They are orally bioavailable and concentrate within the kidney, prostate and lung. Main adverse effects are gastrointestinal disturbance, skin rashes, headache and dizziness. **Ciprofloxacin** inhibits cytochrome P450 and, therefore, interferes with the metabolism of theophylline, which can lead to toxicity in asthmatic subjects.

Rifampin binds to bacterial but not mammalian DNA-dependent RNA polymerase and prevents transcription of mRNA. It has broad-spectrum activity and is a very effective antituberculosis agent. It can enter phagocytic cells and kill intracellular microorganisms. It is orally bioavailable and distributes to body tissues, crosses the blood–brain barrier and is metabolized in the liver. Rifampin induces cytochrome P450, resulting in increased metabolism of glucocorticosteroids, oral contraceptives, phenytoin, barbiturates, ketoconazole, ciclosporin and warfarin. Adverse effects include gastrointestinal disturbance, fever and jaundice. Rifampin is available for the treatment of *Mycobacterium tuberculosis* but drug resistance can develop and is used in combination with isoniazid, ethambutol and pyrazinamide.

Metronidazole is an antiprotozoal agent that is active against anaerobic bacteria. Nitroreductase is produced in anaerobosis, which reduces metronidazole to a short-lived active intermediary that binds to and inhibits the synthesis of DNA. Metronidazole is orally bioavailable and active against *Bacteroides fragilis* (bacterial vaginosis) and *Clostridium difficile*. Metronidazole is a potential carcinogen but the general consensus is that the benefit of treatment outweighs any potential risk.

Antifolates block synthesis of folic acid, an essential cofactor for synthesis of purines and DNA. While humans can utilize external folic acid, bacteria cannot (Fig. 3.43.1B) and antifolates are broad-spectrum bacteriostatic drugs. Sulphonamides (e.g. **sulfamethoxazole**) inhibit dihydrofolate synthetase and **trimethoprim** inhibits dihydrofolate reductase. Resistance to sulphonamides is common, occurring through synthesis of a dihydrofolate synthetase that has lower affinity for sulphonamides, and this resistance is transmitted in Gram-negative bacteria by plasmids. The antifolates are orally bioavailable and used as combination therapy (**cotrimoxazole**: sulfamethoxazole and trimethoprim) for the treatment of urinary tract infections, respiratory infections and against *Pneumocystis carinii*, which causes pneumonia in immunodeficient patients. Adverse reactions to sulphonamides include hypersensitivity reaction (Stevens–Johnson syndrome) and crystalluria.

44. Chemotherapy: antibiotics targeting protein synthesis

Questions
- How are proteins synthesized in bacteria?
- Which drugs target specific steps of protein synthesis?

Agents affecting protein synthesis

Bacterial protein synthesis occurs on ribosomes, which are made up of two subunits (50S and 30S in bacteria). Messenger RNA (mRNA) is the template for protein synthesis and transfer RNA (tRNA) brings each amino acid to the ribosome for assembly into the protein molecule (Fig. 3.44.1). A number of different classes of drug selectively target different elements of this process. These agents are bacteriostatic, with the exception of aminoglycosides and oxazolidinones.

Tetracyclines. These agents selectively enter bacteria by an uptake process and interfere with protein synthesis by reversibly binding to the 30S subunit, impairing the ability of tRNA to attach to mRNA and thus preventing delivery of an amino acid to the growing peptide chain. Tetracyclines have a broad spectrum of activity, although many strains of bacteria are increasingly becoming resistant. The active concentration of tetracycline within bacteria is reduced by the expression of transporters that pump the antibiotic out

of the bacteria. This resistance is transmitted by plasmids and, since the genes that confer resistances are located in close proximity, resistance can also develop to other antibiotics (e.g. sulphonamides). Tetracyclines are orally bioavailable but absorption is impaired by antacids and drinks containing Ca^{2+} and iron owing to the chelating ability of the tetracyclines. Adverse events include gastrointestinal disturbances and, because of their Ca^{2+}-chelating action, they have a tendency to accumulate in growing bone and teeth. They are best avoided by pregnant women, breastfeeding women and in children.

Aminoglycosides. These agents selectively enter aerobic bacteria by an oxygen-dependent transport system. Hence, anaerobic bacteria have a natural resistance. Aminoglycosides bind to the 30S subunit in an irreversible manner, which leads to misreading of mRNA. These agents have a broad spectrum of activity, with the exception of anerobes, streptococci and pnenumococci. Their bactericidal activity can be enhanced when coadministered with penicillins as damage to the cell wall facilitates penetration of aminoglycosides into the bacteria. Resistance to these drugs is an increasing problem. Aminoglycosides have poor oral bioavailability and are administered i.v. **Gentamicin** is the aminoglycoside most commonly used to treat infections by

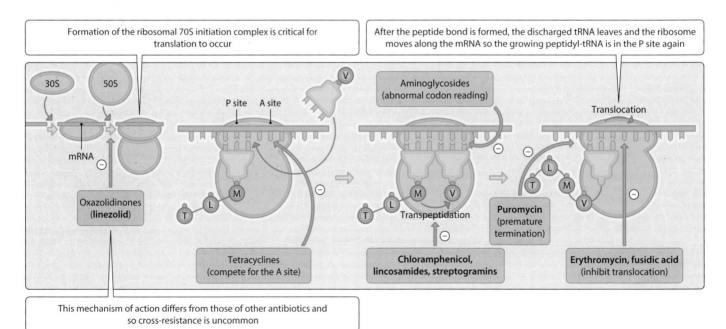

Fig. 3.44.1 Antibiotics acting on protein synthesis.

Gram-negative bacteria, although **tobramycin** is preferred for infection with *Pseudomonas aeruginosa*. **Streptomycin** is used in the treatment of *Mycobacterium tuberculosis*. The side-effects of this drug class limit its utility. Adverse events include ototoxicity: a progressive damage to the sensory cells of the cochlea and vestibular organ of the ear resulting in ataxia, loss of balance, vertigo and deafness. Damage to the kidney renal tubules leads to nephrotoxicity, which will impair plasma clearance of the antibiotic. A rare but serious toxic condition is paralysis of skeletal muscle caused by inhibition of Ca^{2+} uptake into cholinergic nerves and inhibition of release of acetylcholine.

Chloramphenicol is bacteriostatic and binds to the 50S subunit, inhibiting peptidyl transferase activity. This prevents transpeptidation of the growing amino acid chain on the P site to the newly arrived peptidyl tRNA on the A site. This antibiotic has a broad spectrum of activity; however, susceptibility to resistance is high because of expression of 'chloramphenicol acetyltransferase'. The ability of chloramphenicol to cause aplastic anaemia (decreased production of red blood cells) when administered systemically limits its usefulness and it is reserved for life-threatening infections.

Macrolides. Reversible binding of macrolides to the 50S subunit inhibits translocation of peptidyl-tRNA. They have bacteriostatic/bactericidal activity against Gram-positive bacteria and are orally bioavailable or administered parenterally. They have similar activity to penicillin and can be used as an alternative in penicillin-sensitive subjects. Macrolides are used in the treatment of pneumonia (Legionnaires disease, mycoplasma pneumonia) and infections produced by streptococci and staphylococci. Macrolides do not cross the blood–brain barrier. Side-effects include gastrointestinal disturbance, skin rashes, fever and jaundice, the last in treatment of longer than 2 weeks.

Lincosamides. Lincosamides have a similar mechanism of action to macrolides, inhibiting the early elongation of the peptide chain, and are active against Gram-positive bacteria including streptococci, staphylococci and anaerobic bacteria. **Clindamycin** is structurally unrelated to macrolides and chloramphenicol but all three bind to the same site in the 50S subunit and, therefore, can interfere with the binding of each other. Clindamycin is used for staphylococcal infections of the joints and bones and topically in the eye for staphylococcal conjunctivitis. It can be administered orally, parenterally or as a topical cream. It does not cross the blood–brain barrier. Adverse events include gastrointestinal disturbance and the potential to cause enteritis by *Clostridium difficile* but this can be treated with vancomycin and metronidazole.

Streptogramins. These prevent elongation of the peptide chain by inhibiting the peptidyl transferase catalytic centre of the 50S ribosome, thus preventing substrate attachment to the A and P sites. **Quinupristin** and **dalfopristin** are members of this family and individually exhibit modest antibacterial activity. However, they are very effective against infections with staphylococci, streptococci and against vancomycin-resistant *Enterococcus faecalis* and methicillin-resistant *Staphylococcus aureus* when combined (3:7, respectively). They are also used against catheter-related infections, endocarditis, bacteraemia and soft-tissue infections. Streptogramins are administered i.v.; local adverse effects include pain, oedema and inflammation and so they should be infused by a central venous catheter. Other adverse events include nausea, vomiting, diarrhoea and skin rashes. While these drugs are not metabolized by the liver, they do inhibit cytochrome P450 3A4 and this will increase the plasma levels of a number of drugs, including ciclosporin, midazolam and nifedipine.

Oxazolidinones. **Linezolid** is a synthetic antimicrobial agent that is structurally unrelated to other antibiotic agents and has a novel mechanism of action that prevents the formation of the 70S initiation complex and protein synthesis. Linezolid is effective against Gram-positive bacteria and resistant strains (e.g. methicillin-resistant *S. aureus*, vancomycin-resistant enterococci and penicillin-resistant *Streptococcus pneumoniae*). This drug is administered orally or i.v. and side-effects include diarrhoea, headache, nausea and reduced platelet and neutrophil number. These haematological changes should be monitored if the drug is prescribed for prolonged use.

45. Chemotherapy: antiviral drugs

Questions
- What are the drug targets for antiviral agents?
- What are examples of different classes of antiviral drug?

Viruses are intracellular organisms that invade eukaryotic cells by binding to host membrane structures and replicate by inserting their genetic material into the host's genome (Fig. 3.45.1). Because viruses share much of the metabolic machinery of the host cell, it is difficult to find drugs that are specific for the virus. Drugs target attachment or entry into host cells, inhibition of viral transcription, protein synthesis and viral exit from cells (Fig. 3.45.2). Certain drugs are specific for a particular virus:

- herpes simplex: aciclovir, valaciclovir, penciclovir, famciclovir
- varicella-zoster: aciclovir, valaciclovir, famciclovir
- cytomegalovirus: aciclovir, valaciclovir, ganciclovir, foscarnet
- hepatitis B virus: lamivudine
- hepatitis C virus: tribavarin (ribavirin)
- HIV: see Ch. 46.

Inhibition of viral entry

Aminoadamantanes. **Amantadine** and **rimantadine** are 10 carbon ring cyclic structures that inhibit the replication of influenza A viruses by blocking the viral M2 protein ion channel and thereby reducing the effect of this protein on viral uncoating. Amantadine is orally bioavailable and eliminated by renal excretion. As a result, plasma concentrations in older adults will be higher owing to decline in renal function, and side-effects of nausea, anorexia and neurological dysfunction are more prevalent. Rimantadine is also orally bioavailable and hydroxylated in the liver, and older patients with a decline in hepatic function will require lower dosing. Side-effects are similar to amantadine.

Immunoglobulins. Immunoglobulins specific for antigenic determinants on cell surface viral protein can bind and neutralize the ability of virus to infect host cells and improve clearance of the virus from the host. Examples include human normal immunoglobulin (gamma globulin) and immunoglobulins that recognize specific viruses (antihepatitis B).

Inhibition of viral transcription

2′-Deoxyguanosine analogues. These drugs are DNA chain terminators that prevent the formation of viral DNA and inhibit viral DNA polymerase. Antiviral agents like aciclovir are converted to the monophosphate by thymidine kinase but the viral form of this enzyme is more effective so this conversion only occurs in infected cells. Two subsequent phosphorylation reactions by host kinases form the triphosphate substrate for viral DNA polymerase. The insertion of the drug triphosphate derivative into the growing DNA chain stops synthesis proceeding any further and this is

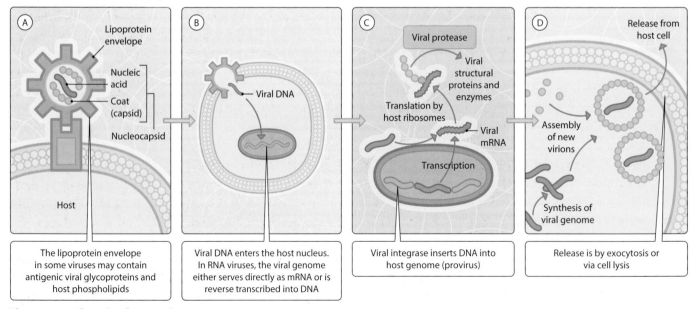

Fig. 3.45.1 Life cycle of a typical virus.

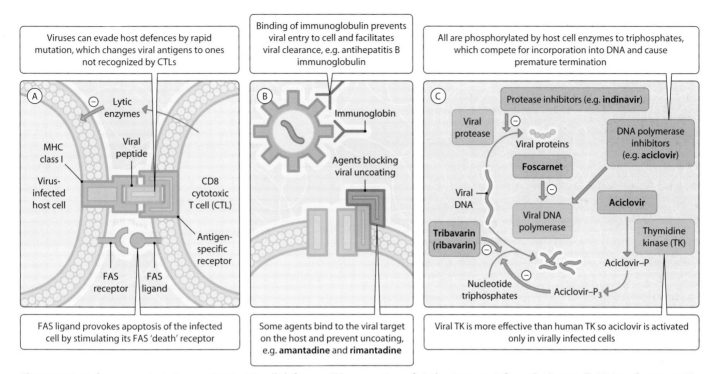

Fig. 3.45.2 Defences against viruses. (A) Host T cell defences; (B) prevention of viral entry or exit from the host cell: (C) interference with viral replication.

irreversible as it cannot be excised by the DNA polymerase-associated 3′,5′-exonuclease. This results in the inactivation of viral DNA polymerase. Aciclovir triphosphate is a significantly more potent inhibitor of viral DNA polymerase than the human enzyme. It is orally bioavailable and excreted unchanged by the kidney. Side-effects are uncommon (crystallization of drug in renal tubules, gastrointestinal disturbances, headache, rash (rare) and encephalopathy (rare)).

Foscarnet. Foscarnet (trisodium phosphonoformate) is an inorganic analogue of pyrophosphate and forms complexes with viral DNA polymerase preventing cleavage of pyrophosphate from nucleoside triphosphates, thus blocking DNA synthesis. It is administered i.v. for cytomegalovirus and aciclovir-resistant herpes simplex viruses. Side-effects include renal insufficiency, nausea and vomiting.

Nucleoside analogues. **Tribavarin** (ribavarin) is a guanosine analogue that is enzymatically converted to the triphosphate in infected cells, thus interfering with viral transcription. It is effective against a range of RNA viruses including Lassa virus (Lassa fever), hantavirus (haemorrhagic fever) and hepatitis C. It undergoes gastrointestinal and liver metabolism and is administered orally, parenterally or intranasally. **Lamivudine** is a pyrimidine analogue that is metabolized intracellularly to lamivudine triphosphate and inhibits hepatitis DNA polymerase and HIV reverse transcriptase. It is orally bioavailable and used in the treatment of hepatitis

B and HIV. Side-effects include anaemia owing to bone marrow suppression.

Immunomodulation

The immune defence against viral infection involves the synthesis and release of interferons α and β from immune cells. These bind to cell surface receptors on infected cells and trigger a cascade of events that protect against viral infection. One of the major actions of interferons is the induction of enzymes in host cells that interfere with the synthesis of viral proteins by inhibiting viral mRNA transcription and translation. **Interferon alfa** is a commercial preparation made using DNA recombinant technology. The interferons are not orally biovailable and must be given i.m. or s.c. They are used to treat infection with hepatitis B, C, papillomavirus and human herpesvirus (Kaposi's sarcoma).

Inhibitors of viral release

Influenza (A and B) leaves infected cells by binding of viral envelope protein haemagglutinin to sialic acid residues of the host target cell receptor. Viral neuraminidase cleaves these sialic acid residues, thereby releasing the virion particles from the cell. A number of neuraminidase inhibitors, **zanamivir** (aerosol) and **oseltamivir** (oral), interfere with the viral replication by inhibiting viral neuraminidase. Virions remain 'tethered' by sialic acid residues to cell surface proteins and each other.

46. Chemotherapy: drugs for HIV

Questions
- Where do drugs target the HIV infective cycle?
- What are the problems with therapy for HIV?

HIV belongs to a family of retroviruses where the genetic information is held as RNA. Consequently, the first step in viral replication is the synthesis of DNA from RNA by viral reverse transcriptase. HIV gains entry to immune system cells by binding to surface proteins (CCR5 on macrophages and dendritic cells; CD4 on T helper cells, macrophages and dendritic cells). The infection eventually destroys the cells of the immune system and at this stage the acquired immunodeficiency syndrome (AIDS) occurs. HIV/AIDS is a major pandemic (although overwhelmingly centred on sub-Saharan Africa, where up to 35% of the adult population is infected with HIV). Because the viral genome can be incorporated into the host genome (a provirus that can be activated at a later date), and can linger in sites less available to drugs (e.g. the brain), it can remain secluded from antiviral actions. Most currently available antiviral agents are only effective while the virus is replicating. There are four major drug classes used in the treatment of HIV with differing targets (Fig. 3.46.1):

- HIV entry into T lymphocytes
- nucleoside inhibition of reverse transcription
- non-nucleoside inhibition of reverse transcription
- protease inhibition.

No one drug is completely effective in HIV and there is the potential for the development of drug resistance. A combination of drug classes, known as highly active antiretroviral therapy (HAART), minimizes this potential. A typical HAART combination would involve two nucleoside reverse transcriptase inhibitors (NRTI) with either a non-nucleoside reverse transcriptase inhibitor (NNRTI) or one or two protease inhibitors. This approach has greatly extended patient survival but the regimen is complex, patient compliance can be an issue and a lifelong commitment to take these medications is required

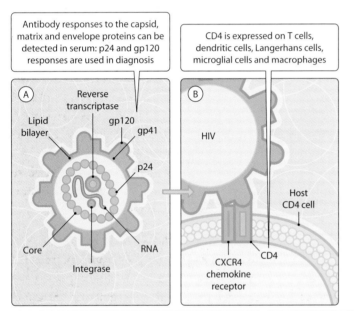

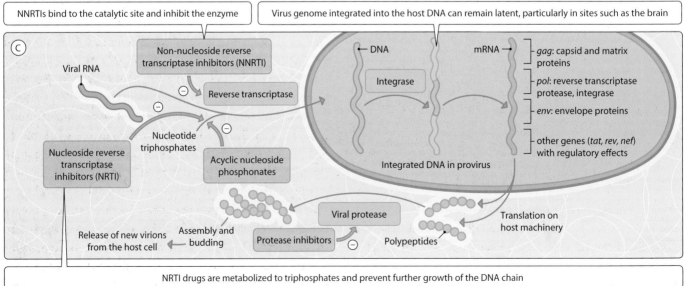

Fig. 3.46.1 Human immunodeficiency virus (HIV). (A) A virion; (B) cell entry; (C) interference with viral replication.

because of the presence of latent virus. There can be unwelcome drug interactions and variations in penetration of drug into reservoir sites such as the brain. In addition the side-effect profile is considerable and drug resistance can still develop.

Inhibition of viral entry (fusion inhibitors)

Fusion inhibitors represent a new class of antiretroviral drug used in the treatment of HIV. **Enfuvirtide** (pentafuside or T20) is a synthetic peptide (36 amino acid residues) that prevents entry into CD4 T lymphocytes. The HIV envelope protein gp120 binds to the CD4 receptor, promoting a conformational change in gp120 and increasing its affinity for T lymphocyte chemokine receptors (CCR5 and CXCR4). This interaction allows a viral membrane glycoprotein (gp41) to form a fusion pore through which viral contents enter the cell. Enfuvirtide binds to specific sites on gp41 and prevents the HIV fusion sequence. The drug is administered s.c. and side-effects of the injection include pain, discomfort, induration and erythema. Peripheral neuropathy and fatigue and increased risk of bacterial pneumonia have been reported. HIV-positive patients who are healthier and who have a less extensive antiretroviral history are most likely to benefit from this treatment.

Inhibition of viral transcription

Nucleoside reverse transcriptase inhibitors

The enzyme reverse transcriptase is a target for a number of drugs, including **zidovudine** (AZT or ZDV), **didanosine** (ddI), **zalcitabine** (ddC), **stavudine** (d4T), **lamivudine** (3TC), **abacavir** (ABC) and **emtricitabine** (FTC). All these dideoxynucleoside inhibitors must be phosphorylated by host cell nucleoside kinases to form the corresponding 5′-triphosphate derivative, which behaves as a chain terminator preventing reverse transcription of viral RNA to DNA. As these derivatives compete with natural substrates for HIV reverse transcriptase, they also behave as competitive inhibitors of this enzyme. NRTIs have considerably lower affinity for host DNA polymerase and, therefore, demonstrate antiviral selectivity. Mutations in reverse transcriptase can produce resistance to these agents, although the development of this resistance can be reduced by using different inhibitors. Adverse effects associated with this drug class are a consequence of non-specific inhibition of mitochondrial DNA polymerases and include myopathy (ZDV), neuropathy (ddI, d4T, ddC) and pancreatitis (ddI).

Non-nucleoside reverse transcriptase inhibitors

The NNRTIs drugs differ from the NRTIs in that they form stable complexes with HIV reverse transcriptase. They bind to a site other than the substrate-binding site by hydrogen bonding. However, resistance develops quite rapidly through mutations in the amino acid residues aligning the NNRTI-binding 'pocket'.

The most common side-effect reported with **nevirapine** and **delavirdine** is rash and with **efavirenz**, CNS complaints such as dizziness.

Acyclic nucleoside phosphonates

Acyclic nucleoside phosphonates possess a phosphonate group attached to the acyclic nucleoside moiety through a stable P–C bond. This has several advantages: it is resistant to cellular esterases (splitting the phosphate P–O–C bond), only two phosphorylation steps are required to produce the active triphosphate and the drug does not depend on the virus-induced thymidine kinase to initiate phosphorylation. This means that the drugs are active against strains that have developed resistance at the thymidine kinase step. Furthermore, they are also not dependent upon the nucleoside kinase reaction that is required for the action of NRTI inhibitors and where resistance can also develop. The triphosphate derivative serves as a chain terminator.

Examples of this drug class include **tenofovir disoproxil fumarate** (HIV), **cidofovir** (cytomegalovirus retinitis) and **adefovir** dipivoxil (hepatitis B). These drugs act as chain terminators for reverse transcriptase reactions (HIV) and DNA polymerase (DNA viruses) as they become irreversibly incorporated into DNA. Adverse reactions include Fanconi's syndrome (phosphate depletion and dysfunction of the renal tubules) caused by increased excretion of phosphate, glucose, amino acids and other intermediary metabolites and which can result in osteomalacia (tenofovir, cidofovir).

Inhibition of protein synthesis

A number of viruses (HIV, herpes) utilize viral proteases to cleave precursor polypeptides into functional proteins. A number of HIV protease inhibitors (**saquinavir, ritonavir, indinavir, nelfinavir, amprenavir, lopinavir, atazanavir**) share the same structural motif that make them resistant to cleavage and hence are inhibitors of viral protease. They have the advantage that they do not require phosphorylation reactions to activate them (as is the case for NRTIs and NNRTIs). However, resistance develops through mutations of the HIV protease. Protease inhibitors are substrates and inhibitors of cytochrome P450 and clinically important drug interactions occur (e.g. proton pump inhibitors, benzodiazepines, histamine H_2 antagonists, statins and warfarin). Common side-effects include nausea, vomiting, dizziness, peripheral neuropathy and rash. This drug class also causes lipodystrophy, which is characterized by altered pattern of fat distribution (wasting of peripheral fat, central accumulation of fat), hyperlipidaemia and insulin resistance. The protease inhibitor atazanavir, the first once a day protease inhibitor, appears to cause fewer lipid abnormalities than other protease inhibitors.

47. Chemotherapy: anthelmintic agents

Questions
- How do anthelmintic agents act?
- What are examples of different classes of anthelmintic agents?

Parasitic helminths are complex multicellular organisms with nervous systems and organs and a life cycle that involves time spent in more than one host (Fig. 3.47.1). The helminths reproduce sexually in the primary definitive host (usually human but not always) to give rise to eggs or larvae, which then exit the host to continue their life cycle. In human infections, the eggs are distinctive and help to identify the parasite (Fig. 3.47.2). Parasitic helminths that infect humans form three groups: tapeworm (cestodes), roundworms (nematode) and flukes (trematode).

To be effective, an anthelminthic must be able to penetrate the cuticle of the worm or gain access to its alimentary tract. The route and dose is, therefore, important and must be chosen carefully since parasitic worms cannot be relied upon to consume sufficient amounts of the drug for it to be effective. An anthelminthic can act by causing paralysis of the worm or by damaging its cuticle, which can alert the host immune defences to remove the parasite. Drugs that interfere with the metabolism of the worm tend to be highly effective against one type of worm but ineffective against others (Table 3.47.1).

Benzimidazoles. These agents (**thiabendazole**, **mebendazole** and **albendazole**) selectively bind with high affinity to free β-tubulin and inhibit the polymerization and breakdown of cytoskeleton microtubules. This interferes with microtubule-dependent uptake of glucose, a necessary energy source for the parasite. These drugs have considerably greater selectivity for parasitic microtubule function over the mammalian counterpart. **Albendazole** has broad-spectrum activity against nematodes and in the treatment of cestodes. It is orally bioavailable and treatment for 4 weeks is desirable, often two or three times per day. Its absorption is enhanced by fatty meals. Side-effects include abdominal pain, nausea, vomiting, alopecia and neutropenia. These drugs should not be administered to pregnant women as they are teratogenic.

Praziquantel. Praziquantel is an effective broad-spectrum anthelmintic against trematodes and cestodes. It appears to interfere with Ca^{2+} homeostasis, by increasing membrane

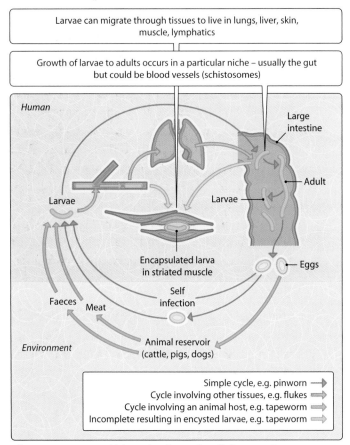

Fig. 3.47.1 General life cycles for multicellular parasites.

Larvae can migrate through tissues to live in lungs, liver, skin, muscle, lymphatics

Growth of larvae to adults occurs in a particular niche – usually the gut but could be blood vessels (schistosomes)

Human

Large intestine

Larvae

Adult

Larvae

Encapsulated larva in striated muscle

Eggs

Self infection

Faeces

Meat

Environment

Animal reservoir (cattle, pigs, dogs)

Simple cycle, e.g. pinworm
Cycle involving other tissues, e.g. flukes
Cycle involving an animal host, e.g. tapeworm
Incomplete resulting in encysted larvae, e.g. tapeworm

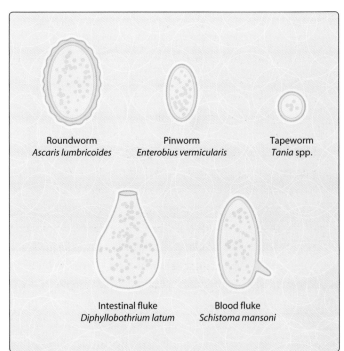

Fig. 3.47.2 Eggs of helminths.

Roundworm
Ascaris lumbricoides

Pinworm
Enterobius vermicularis

Tapeworm
Tania spp.

Intestinal fluke
Diphyllobothrium latum

Blood fluke
Schistoma mansoni

Table 3.47.1 DRUGS USED IN HELMINTH INFECTIONS

Helminth	Drug
Cestodes	
Intestinal tapeworms (*Taenia saginata, T. solium*)	Praziquantel, niclosamide
Echinococcus granulosus (hydatid disease)	Albendazole, praziquantel
Hymenolepis nana (hymenolepiasis)	Praziquantel, niclosamide
Nematodes	
Common roundworm (*Ascaris lumbricoides*)	Albendazole, pyrantel, levamisole
Threadworm (pinworm) (*Enterobius vermicularis*)	Albendazole, pyrantel
Hookworm (*Necator* spp.)	Albendazole, pyrantel
Strongyloides stercoralis (called threadworm in the USA)	Albendazole, ivermectin
Wuchereria bancrofti, Loa loa (roundworm; filariasis)	Diethylcarbamazine, ivermectin
Trichinella spiralis (trichiniasis)	Thiabendazole
Onchocerca volvulus (river blindness)	Ivermectin
Trematodes	
Blood flukes (*Schistosoma* spp.)	Praziquantel, oxamniquine
Lung, intestinal flukes	Praziquantel
Liver fluke (*Fasciola hepaticus*)	Praziquantel

permeability to Ca^{2+}. Contraction of the parasite ensues, resulting in paralysis. Dying parasites detach from the tissues and may be destroyed by the host's immune system. The drug is administered three times daily for up to 2 days, with side-effects including headache, dizziness, drowsiness and abdominal discomfort. Praziquantel undergoes extensive first pass metabolism and oral bioavailability is reduced further by concomitant use of antiepileptic drugs (phenytoin, carbamazepine), which induce cytochrome P450. In contrast, cimetidine, which inhibits cytochrome P450 activity, will reduce the metabolism of praziquantel and so increase plasma concentrations after oral dosing.

Ivermectin. Ivermectin is an extremely potent broad-spectrum anthelmintic drug used in the control of nematode infections in animals and against onchocerciasis (river blindness) in humans. Ivermectin is derived from the soil mould *Streptomyces avermitilis* and potentiates the opening of GABA-gated chloride-sensitive channels. This results in hyperpolarization of nerve and muscle cells, causing tonic paralysis of the nematode's muscle system and death. Repeated dosing for up to a year may be required where the disease is endemic to reduce microfilariae number. The appearance of dermatitis and ocular disease are significantly reduced. Side-effects arise from the host's reaction to the dying microfilariae and include pruritus, rash, dizziness and oedema of the face and limbs. Selectivity for parasitic over mammalian chloride-gated ion channel is achieved by choice of dosage and because GABA receptors are found in the mammalian CNS and ivermectin does not readily cross the blood–brain barrier. In other filariases, including *Wuchereria bancrofti, Burgia malayi* and *Loa loa*, ivermectin is active against blood-borne microfilariae but ineffective against adult worms in the lymphatic system. It is also used in the treatment of scabies and head lice.

Diethylcarbamazine. The mode of action of this drug is not entirely understood but it kills both microfilariae and adult worms and, therefore, remains the drug of choice for *W. bancrofti, B. malayi* and *L. loa*. Side-effects include gastrointestinal disturbances, headache and the host's reaction to damaged or dead parasites including skin reactions, dizziness and tachycardia.

Niclosamide. Niclosamide is a salicylamide derivative and is used in the treatment of tapeworm infection. The drug damages the end of the worm that attaches to the gastrointestinal tract, resulting in expulsion. Niclosamide is relatively safe as it is not absorbed across the gastrointestinal tract.

Piperazine. Anthelmintic action against common roundworm and threadworm infections occurs through action as a GABA receptor agonist at the parasitic neuromuscular junction. This causes paralysis and leads to expulsion of the parasite from the host. Selectivity for the parasitic GABA-gated chloride channel is achieved since this receptor is only found within the CNS of mammals. Piperazine is given orally and is poorly absorbed. Side-effects are limited but include gastrointestinal disturbance and, in some instances, dizziness and incoordination.

Pyrantel. This drug can be used against pinworm (e.g. *Enterobius vermicularis*) and most nematode infections. It selectively causes depolarization of muscle cells, possible via activation of nematode nicotine receptors, thereby inducing paralysis.

Levamisole. This drug has been used to treat gastrointestinal nematodes. Like pyrantel, it causes muscle paralysis in the parasite by activating nicotinic receptors at the neuromuscular junction.

48. Chemotherapy: antiprotozoan agents

Questions
- What are the drug targets for antiprotazoan agents?
- What are examples of different classes of antiprotozoan agents?

There are four major groups of protozoal parasites: sporozoates, flagellates, ciliates and amoebae. Unlike helminths, protozoa are single cell organisms that rapidly divide in the infected host.

Malaria

Malaria is transmitted by the *Anopheles* mosquito, which carries sporozoites of *Plasmodium* spp. that infect the human host when a mosquito bites (Fig. 3.48.1). The parasites infect liver cells and begin asexual division before being released into the blood as merozoites, which invade and multiply within red blood cells. Cell lysis releases the parasite into the bloodstream and gives rise to the clinical symptoms of malaria. Alternatively, some merozites differentiate into male and female gametocytes, which reenter a mosquito that bites an infected host and thus continue the parasite's life cycle. *P. falciparum* causes the most deaths from malaria. A number of different drugs are available for the treatment of this disease (Table 3.48.1).

4-Aminoquinolines and aryl amino alcohols. This drug class is structurally derived from quinine, the active constituent of the *Cinchona* bark. These drugs (e.g. **chloroquine**) inhibit haem polymerase, the parasite enzyme that converts free haem, released from the degradation of haemoglobin in the red blood cell, to insoluble crystals (haemozoin) thus protecting the parasite from the oxidizing effects of free haem. Drugs in this class include **amodiaquine** although its use is limited because of its side-effect of agranulocytosis (but it is of use in chloroquine-resistant parasites). **Mefloquine** and **halofantrine** are also effective in resistant strains but can cause unwanted neuropsychiatric and arrhythmic effects, respectively. **Lumefantrine** is used in combination with **artemether** (**co-artemether**) and is not associated with neurological side-effects, although is susceptible to cross-resistance with mefloquine. Side-effects of the aryl amino alcohols include cinchonism (tinnitus, hearing loss, nausea, restlessness).

8-Aminoquinolines. **Primaquine** has long been used for the eradication of the liver stages in *P. vivax* infection and killing gametocytes of *P. falciparum*. One of the major adverse reactions to this treatment is the induction of haemolytic anaemia in subjects with a deficiency in glucose-6-phosphate dehydrogenase, which can be life threatening. **Tafenoquine** is a derivative of primaquine that has a longer half-life and so requires less-frequent dosing. Haemolytic anaemia is still a distinct possibility.

Antifolates. Unlike humans, the malarial parasite is required to synthesize folates, which are used in the synthesis of nucleotides required for DNA transcription. The combination **sulfadoxine–pyrimethamine** is a most effective treatment of malaria. The antifolates inhibit folate production by inhibiting dihydropteroate synthase (type I antifolate; sulphonamides (**sulfadoxine**, **sulfalene**), **dapsone**) and dihydrofolate reductase (type II antifolate;

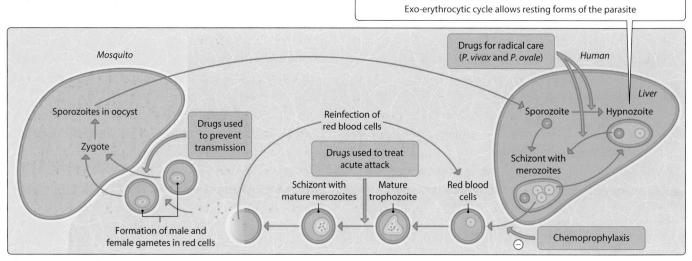

Fig. 3.48.1 The life cycle of the malarial parasite and site of action of drugs (see Table 3.48.1).

Table 3.48.1 ACTION OF ANTIMALARIAL DRUGS

Stage	Effect	Drugs
Merozoites	Block the link between the exoerythrocytic and erythrocytic stages (chemoprophylactic)	4-Aminoquinolines, antifolates, antibiotics, arteminsin
Erythrocytic forms	Can cure *P. falciparum* or *P. malariae* infections as these have no exoerythrocytic stage; suppress acute attack for *P. vivax* or *P. ovale* but the exoerythrocytic forms can cause later relapses	Quinoline-methanols, 4-aminoquinolines, halofantrine, arteminsin derivatives, antibiotics, antifolates
Tissue schizonts	Effect a radical cure by acting on the parasites in the liver	8-Aminoquinoline (primaquine), antibiotic (tetracycline), antifolates
Gametocytes	Reduce the spread of infection	8-Aminoquinoline (primaquine), arteminsin derivatives

pyrimethamine, **proguanil**, **chlorproguanil**). This drug group inhibits the growing stages of the parasite when used in combination for the prophylactic treatment of malaria. Hypersensitivity to the sulphonamide component gives rise to epidermal necrosis (Steven–Johnson syndrome).

Arteminsin derivatives.   The sesquiterpene arteminsin is an active product of *Artemisia annua* with potent antimalarial activity. The release of haem within the food vacuole reacts with peroxide moiety in arteminsin. The ensuing generation of oxygen radicals is damaging to the parasite. Several semisynthetic derivatives, including **artemether**, **arteether** and **artesunate**, show good efficacy against malaria. They have a faster onset of action than conventional antimalarial agents and reduce blood parasite levels and associated symptoms. They are active against gametocytes, which reinfect *Anopheles* mosquito. Combination with other antimalarial agents (e.g. artesunate and mefloquine) reduces the risk of resistance. This drug class appears to be safe despite evidence of neurotoxic and embryotoxic effects in animals at high doses. It can be administered rectally in small children.

Antibiotics.   During its evolution, the malarial parasite acquired an organelle (apicoplast) that contains the appropriate machinery for replication and serves an important metabolic role. Antibiotics that inhibit protein synthesis within the apicoplast (tetracyclines, macrolides, lincosamides) and mitochondrial protein synthesis of the parasite (tetracyclines) are used in prophylaxis of malaria. The onset of action is slow and it is usual to combine antibiotics with other antimalarial agents (e.g. doxycycline and artesunate). Clindamycin provides an alternative to doxycycline as the latter is responsible for photosensitizing reactions and is contraindicated in small children and pregnant women.

New antimalarial drugs.   Combination of lumefantrine (aryl amino alcohol) with artemether (co-artemether) has proven efficacy in the treatment of malaria. Similarly, a combination of atovaquone and proguanil is also used. Atovoquone inhibits mitochondrial electron transport via the cytochrome *c* reductase complex; the combination with proguanil reduces the risk of resistance and is synergistic. The combination chlorproguanil–dapsone is intended to be used as a replacement for sulfadoxine–pyrimethamine and is currently undergoing clinical trials. This combination offers the advantage of reducing the risk of emergence of resistance as both drugs have a relatively short plasma half-life. **Pyronaridine** is a 4-aminoquinoline derivative and is active against chloroquine-resistant malaria.

Other protozoan diseases

Other protozoal infections include trypanosomiasis, leismaniasis, giardiasis, toxoplasmosis, trichomoniasis and pneumocytosis, for which there are a number of pharmacological treatments.

Pneumocystis carinii (now *P. jiroveci*).   This organism has structural features of both protozoa and fungi and its precise classification is unclear. It is widely distributed in the animal kingdom without causing disease, but it now causes opportunistic infection in immunodeficient patients; *P. jiroveci* pneumonia is often the presenting symptom for onset of AIDS and is a leading cause of death. Drugs used include **cotrimoxazole**, **pentamidine**, **trimethoprim–dapsone**.

Entamoeba histolytica.   Amoebiasis is caused by ingestion of cysts of this organism; the cysts develop in the intestine into trophozoites that invades the submucosa, leading either acutely to dysentery or to a chronic intestinal infection without dysentery. The parasite may also invade the liver, leading to the development of liver abscesses. Choice of drug depends largely on the site and type of infection and includes **metronidazole**, **tinidazole** and **diloxanide**.

49. Chemotherapy: antifungal agents

Questions
- What are the drug targets for antifungal agents?
- What are the different classes of antifungal agent?

Unlike plants, fungi do not have chlorophyll and, therefore, have evolved to live as saprophytes or parasites and reproduce by spores. Fungi can be pathogenic (*Candida albicans, Aspergillus fumigatus, Cryptococcus neoformans*) or non-pathogenic (*Saccharomyces cerevisiae*). Yeasts are round and unicellular and multiply by budding or fission. There are also filamental forms made up of long tubes known as hyphae. A collection of hyphae is a mycelium, which is vegetative but if it is growing on a surface it can produce aerial extensions that carry spores. The dimorphic fungi can exist as yeasts or filaments and it is usually the yeast form that occurs in tissues and the filamentous form in the environment. *Candida* spp., however, form a mycelium in tissues. A number of drug classes have been developed that target fungal envelope (wall and membrane), microtubule assembly and DNA synthesis (Fig. 3.49.1). Fungal infections can damage tissues in several ways (Fig. 3.49.2).

Cell envelope

Polyene macrolides. Ergosterol is the principal sterol in the fungal membrane phospholipid bilayer, whereas the mammalian membrane contains cholesterol. **Amphotericin B** and **nystatin** bind to ergosterol, causing it to change its conformation, which results in the destabilization of the fungal membrane, leading to leakage of intracellular contents and fungicidal action. Amphotericin B and nystatin have greater affinity for ergosterol (cylindrical structure than cholesterol (sigmoidal structure), which is the basis of the relative selectivity of these agents for fungal cells. Amphotericin B has a broad spectrum of activity but is poorly absorbed from the gastrointestinal tract, which may be of advantage for the treatment of gastrointestinal infections or topically for dermatological conditions. It can be administered as a slow infusion for systemic use but it is associated with nephrotoxicity; this can be minimized by changes to the formulation (e.g. encapsulating the drug in liposomes) so that the levels of amphotericin B reaching the kidney are reduced. Other side-effects include fever, chills, hypotension, vomiting and headaches. **Nystatin** is used topically or orally for gastrointestinal infections. **Natamycin**

and **candicidin** are used in the treatment of ocular and vaginal fungal infections.

'Azoles' (imidazoles and triazoles) bind to the iron core of the haem moiety of fungal cytochrome P450 lanosterol 14α-demethylase, is critical for the synthesis of ergosterol. As a result, unusual sterols are synthesized and incorporated into fungal membranes, disrupting its integrity and the function of membrane-bound enzymes. The imidazole class is mainly used for topical application, although **ketoconazole** has oral bioavailability. Side-effects include nausea and vomiting. Importantly, ketoconazole inhibits steroid biosynthesis, resulting in endocrine abnormalities (e.g. decreased libido, gynaecomastia, menstrual irregularities) and hepatotoxicity. It is best avoided in pregnant and breastfeeding women. Inhibition of P450 enzymes by ketoconazole increases plasma levels of certain drugs (e.g. warfarin), and vice versa. The absorption of azoles is reduced by antacids, cimetidine or rifampin and increased by thiazide diuretics. Triazoles are used for systemic infections; while some show greater selectivity for

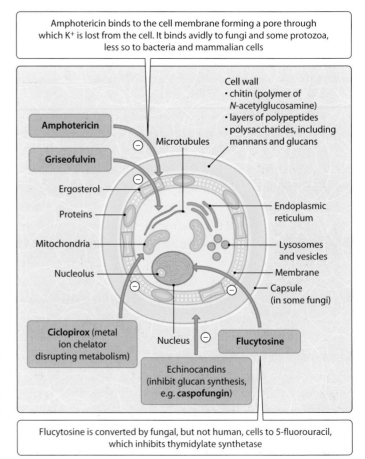

Amphotericin binds to the cell membrane forming a pore through which K⁺ is lost from the cell. It binds avidly to fungi and some protozoa, less so to bacteria and mammalian cells

Cell wall
- chitin (polymer of N-acetylglucosamine)
- layers of polypeptides
- polysaccharides, including mannans and glucans

Amphotericin

Griseofulvin

Microtubules

Ergosterol

Proteins

Endoplasmic reticulum

Mitochondria

Lysosomes and vesicles

Nucleolus

Membrane

Capsule (in some fungi)

Ciclopirox (metal ion chelator disrupting metabolism)

Nucleus

Flucytosine

Echinocandins (inhibit glucan synthesis, e.g. **caspofungin**)

Flucytosine is converted by fungal, but not human, cells to 5-fluorouracil, which inhibits thymidylate synthetase

Fig. 3.49.1 Drug targets.

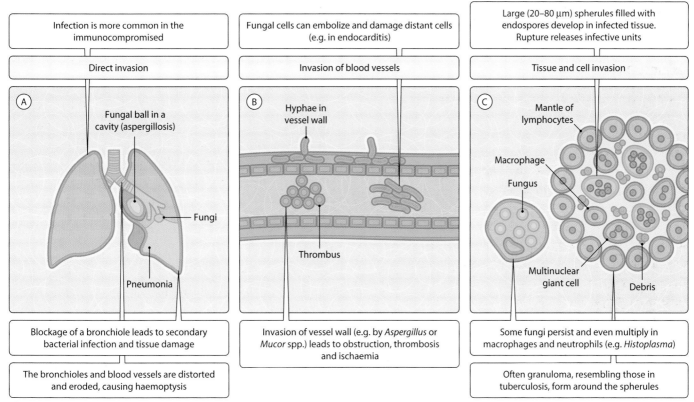

Fig. 3.49.2 Tissue damage by fungal infection.

fungal cytochrome P450 (e.g. **voriconazole**, **posaconazole**), others (e.g. **imidazole**, **fluconazole**) have human P450 actions that increase levels of other drugs. Fluconazole is almost totally absorbed orally and is used in the treatment of candidiasis, cryptococcosis and other mycoses.

The enzyme squalene 2,3-epoxidase is involved in the biosynthesis of ergosterol and its inhibition by allylamines leads to squalene accumulation in the cell wall and fungal death. **Terbinafine** and **naftifine** against filamentous fungi (e.g. moulds) and very few pathogenic yeasts. Terbinafine is orally active and because of its lipophilicity concentrates in the dermis and epidermis and is used for the topical treatment of ringworm athletes foot and onychomycosis (nail infection). Side-effects include nausea, loss of taste and allergic skin reactions.

The drug **amorolfine** inhibits two enzymes involved late in the biosynthesis of ergosterol and is used as topical treatment as a lacquer (e.g. onychomycosis in the nails). Application directly to the skin is ineffective because nail keratin is somewhat impermeable.

The echinocardins represent a new class of antifungal agent. **Capsofungin** is a semisynthetic molecule from the fungus *Glarea lozoyenesis*. It inhibits the enzyme β(1,3)-glycan synthase and the biosynthesis of β(1,3)-glycan polysaccharides, an essential component of the fungal cell wall. This agent has a broad spectrum of activity, is fungicidal and fungistatic and is specific for fungi. Caspofungin is given i.v. and inhibits infection by filamentous fungi (*Aspergillus* spp.) and yeasts (*Candida* spp.). Side-effects include fever, headache and nausea.

Microtubule assembly

Griseofulvin is an antifungal agent isolated from *Penicillium griseofulvum*. Its precise mechanism of action is not known but it is thought to interfere with microtubule assembly and mitosis. It is administered orally, binds to keratin and concentrates in the skin and, therefore, is mainly used to treat ringworm and athlete's foot. Side-effects include hepatoxicity, hypersensitivity reaction (characterized by rash, neutropenia, fever), headache, irritability and photosensitivity. Griseofulvin also induces P450, thereby causing drug interactions.

DNA synthesis

Flucytosine (5-flurocytosine) is converted to the active metabolite 5-fluorouracil within susceptible fungi and is incorporated into RNA, and inhibits protein synthesis. 5-Fluorouracil is also converted to a potent inhibitor of thymidylate synthase, thus affecting DNA synthesis. Resistance can develop and so it is used in combination with other antifungal agents (e.g. amphotericin B). It is orally bioavailable and penetrates cerebrospinal fluid. Adverse events include hepatotoxicity, hair loss and bone marrow suppression.

50. Chemotherapy: anticancer agents

Questions
■ What do anticancer agents target?
■ What are examples of different classes of anticancer agents?

Chemotherapy for cancer can be used in isolation or as an adjunct to other forms of therapy. Compared with bacterial disease, cancer presents a difficult problem in that cancer cells and normal cells are similar in many respects. Consequently, it is more difficult to find general, exploitable, biochemical differences between them. Cancer cells differ from normal cells in four ways:

■ uncontrolled proliferation
■ loss of function because of failure to differentiate
■ invasiveness
■ ability to metastasize.

The drugs used in cancer therapy target the cellular mechanisms of uncontrolled proliferation and many target the ability of cells to divide (Fig. 3.50.1). Most anticancer drugs will also affect rapidly dividing normal cells and so are likely to have unwanted effects of depression of bone marrow and growth, impairment of healing, hair loss, sterility and teratogenicity. Many cause nausea and vomiting.

Alkylating agents
One of the major classes of drug used in the treatment of cancer are agents that directly alkylate DNA, including nitrogen mustards (cyclophosphamide, ifosfamide), nitrosoureas (lomustine, carmustine) and others (cisplatin, busulphan, dacarbazine), thereby impairing DNA synthesis and cell division (Fig. 3.50.1). Some require enzymatic conversion (e.g. cyclosphosphamide, ifosfamide and dacarbazine) or spontaneous conversion (e.g. lomustine) to an active alkylating metabolite. They have a preferential activity on rapidly proliferating cells and are not cell cycle specific. However, as the cell enters S phase, the presence of damaged DNA (in this case alkylated) signals cell cycle arrest and cell death. Side-effects of cytotoxic drugs include myelosuppression, alopecia, inhibited proliferation of gastrointestinal epithelium and fertility effects.

Cytotoxic antibiotics
A number of antibacterial agents intercalate with DNA, resulting in numerous DNA strand breaks. They also form complexes with topoisomerase II and generate oxygen radicals, which also facilitate strand breakage and cell cycle arrest. Side-effects are the same as for direct acting alkylating agents. Examples include dactinomycin (binds DNA) **bleomycin** (DNA fragmentation), **plicamycin** (similar to dactinomycin),

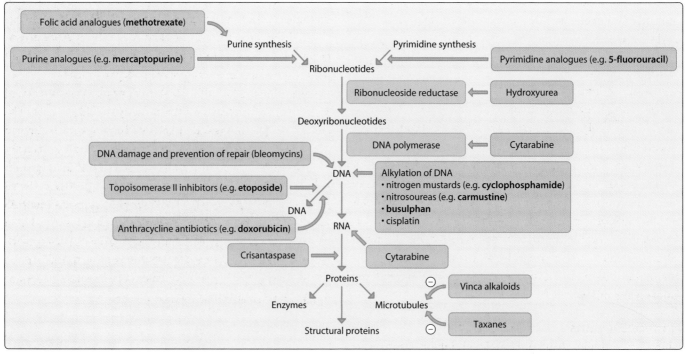

Fig. 3.50.1 Summary of sites of action of cytotoxic drugs.

mitomycin (cross-links DNA) and **doxorubicin** (binds DNA, inhibits RNA and DNA synthesis, topoisomerase inhibitor).

Topoisomerase inhibitors

Topoisomerase is an enzyme critical for resealing of DNA strand breaks. Drugs that target this enzyme (e.g. **etoposide**, **doxorubicin**) result in DNA strand breaks that are not repaired, leading to cell cycle arrest. These agents work predominantly during the S phase of the cell cycle. Side-effects are similar to alkylating agents.

Antimetabolites

A number of agents interfere with the biosynthesis of nucleotides essential for the synthesis of DNA or are incorporated into DNA, thereby impairing DNA synthesis (Fig. 3.50.2A). **Methotrexate** inhibits dihydrofolate reductase, an enzyme essential for the formation of tetrahydrofolate from dihydrofolate. Tetrahydrofolate is needed for the de novo synthesis of thymidine, which is required for DNA synthesis and methotrexate is, therefore, active during S phase in rapidly proliferating cells and cancerous cells. Similarly, pyrimidine analogues including **5-fluorouracil** are phosphorylated and incorporated into DNA in place of thymidylate, thereby interfering with DNA synthesis. These analogues also inhibit thymidylate synthetase and impair RNA processing. Nucleoside analogues of cytosine (e.g. **cytarabine**) are phosphorylated and incorporated into DNA, thereby terminating chain extension. A variety of purine analogues including **mercaptopurine** and **thioguanine** inhibit the de novo synthesis of purines, which are important precursors of DNA, and may also be phosphorylated and incorporated into DNA. Side-effects are similar to alkylating agents.

Mitotic agents

A number of substances bind to and inactivate tubulin, a protein critical for the formation of microtubule assembly. These microtubules are necessary for cytoskeletal function but more importantly for nuclear and cell division during the G2–M phase. Vinca alkaloids (e.g. **vincristine**, **vinblastine**) prevent polymerization or the association of tubulin monomers. Side-effects are similar to those with alkylating agents but these drugs are also neurotoxic, although this is less of a problem for **vinorelbine**. Taxanes (**paclitaxel**, **docetaxel**) promote microtubule assembly. These drugs bind to tubulin and prevent microtubule disassembly, thus interfering with normal cell function and mitosis.

Hormonal agents

Glucocorticosteroids (e.g. prednisolone) inhibit lymphocyte proliferation and are used for leukaemia and lymphoma.

Tamoxifen (anti-oestrogen) is a partial oestrogen agonist that blocks the tumour-promoting action of oestrogen in mammary cells by binding to the oestrogen receptor. It is used in postmenopausal women with oestrogen receptor-positive breast cancer. The small incidence of uterine cancer and thromboembolism has led to the development of aromatase inhibitors (e.g. formestane) for the treatment of postmenopausal breast cancer.

Gonadotrophin-releasing hormone (GnRH) analogues (e.g. **goserelin**) reduce androgen synthesis and are used to treat breast and prostate cancer. They are administered s.c. and side-effects include impotence, decreased libido, gynaecomastia, fluid retention and bone demineralization.

Anti-androgens (e.g. **flutamide**) block the cellular actions of androgens and are orally bioavailable for the treatment of prostate cancer. They initially induce a compensatory rise in LH and give rise to a testosterone surge (flare). This can be prevented by combined therapy with a GnRH agonist. Side-effects include nausea, vomiting and diarrhoea.

Biological agents

Targeting specific proteins essential for tumour growth, survival and metastasis can be effective strategy in breast, lung and colon cancer and is being actively pursued for other forms of cancer. The advantage is that the side-effects associated with cytotoxic chemotherapy are reduced. Some monoclonal antibodies target cell surface molecules. **Rituximab** (Rituxan) is a chimeric molecule targeting CD20 on B cells and is used to treat B cell non-Hodgkin lymphoma. The Fc portion of the antibody activates complement and antibody-dependent cytotoxicity of the target cells. **Gemtuzumab ozogamicin** (Mylotarg) targets CD33, delivering a toxin to myeloid blast cells in acute myelogenous leukaemia. **Alemtuzumab** (Campath) targets CD52 on mature lymphocytes in chronic lymphocytic leukaemia.

Other monoclonal antibodies target proteins in cells required for growth and proliferation (particularly tyrosine kinases (TK) and TK receptors). **Trastuzamab** (Herceptin) targets HER2/neu (TK receptor) expressed in metastatic breast cancer, **bevacizumab** (Avastin) targets vascular endothelial growth factor (acts via TK receptors) in metastatic colon cancer. Small molecule inhibitors of TK or TK receptors include **imatinib mesylate** (Gleevac: inhibiting the TKs Bcl–Abl and c-kit in chronic myelogenous leukaemia and non-epithelial gastrointestinal tract tumours, respectively) and **gefitinib** (Iressa: inhibiting the TK domain of epidermal growth factor receptor in metastatic small cell lung cancer).

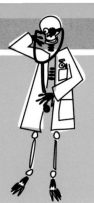

Glossary

Abbreviations

ACE	angiotensin-converting enzyme
AV	atrioventricular
cAMP	cyclic adenosine monophosphate
CD	cluster of differentiation
CNS	central nervous system
COMT	catechol-O-methyltransferase
COX	cyclooxygenase
CYP	cytochrome P450
GABA	gamma-aminobutyric acid
HDL	high density lipoprotein
5HT	5-hydroxytryptamine (serotonin)
i.m.	intramuscular
i.v.	intravenous
LDL	low density lipoprotein
MAO	monoamine oxidase
NSAIDs	non-steroidal anti-inflammatory drugs
SA	sinoatrial
s.c.	subcutaneous
SSRI	serotonin selective reuptake inhibitor

Terms

absorption
the process governing entry of drug into the body

adenylyl cyclase
enzyme that converts adenosine triphosphate into the second messenger, cyclic adenosine monophosphate (cAMP) in cells

affinity
a measure (usually in molar terms) of the strength of binding of a drug to its receptor

agonist
a chemical that binds to specific amino acid sequence on a receptor and stimulates a pharmacological effect

angiotensin-converting enzyme
enzyme expressed on endothelial cells that converts angiotensin I to angiotensin II and metabolizes bradykinin to inactive peptides

antagonist
a chemical that prevents an agonist from inducing a pharmacological effect

autoreceptors
activation of autoreceptors present on presynaptic nerve terminals limits the amount of neurotransmitter released from nerve terminals (negative feedback regulation)

catechol-O-methyltransferase (COMT)
an enzyme found in neuronal and non-neuronal cells that is responsible for the metabolism of catecholamines

chemical antagonist
a chemical that physically binds to an agonist (e.g. chelating agents and neutralizing antibodies)

chemoreceptor trigger zone (CTZ)
a region of the brain stem involved in nausea and vomiting; it responds to hormones, drugs, toxins and receives vagal innervation

chemotherapy
synthetic chemicals used in the treatment of infections and cancer

cyclooxygenase (COX)
enzyme responsible for the conversion of arachidonic acid to cyclic endoperoxides, the precursors for the prostaglandins

cytochrome P450 (CYP)
a family of enzymes predominantly found in the liver that metabolizes drug by oxidation and reduction reactions

depolarization
change in membrane potential (more positive) following an increase in the membrane permeability to Na^+ via cell surface ion channels in excitable cells

desensitization
loss of function following prolonged exposure of receptors to drug

disease-modifying antirheumatoid drugs (DMARD)
a group of chemicals with diverse mechanism of action used in the treatment of rheumatoid arthritis

distribution
the process that governs the presence of drug molecules throughout the total body fluid compartment

EC$_{50}$

the molar concentration of agonist that produces 50% of the maximum pharmacological response for that agonist

ED$_{50}$

the dose of drug that produces 50% of the maximum response in vivo or the dose that produces a specified response in vivo in 50% of subjects

efficacy

a dimensionless property that is a measure of the ability of a drug to induce a conformational change to a receptor and, therefore, produce a pharmacological response

elimination

the process that governs the removal of drug from the body

first pass metabolism

drugs absorbed following oral administration enter the portal circulation and are carried to the liver via the port vein where they are susceptible to metabolism by the liver

full agonist

term used to describe an agonist that produces a maximal pharmacological effect in a given tissue

guanylyl cyclase

enzyme that converts guanosine triphosphate into the second messenger, cyclic guanosine monophosphate (cGMP)

half-life

a pharmacokinetic term that is a measure of disappearance of a chemical: the biological half-life of a drug quantifies the time required for 50% of drug to be cleared from the plasma

hyperpolarization

change in membrane potential (more negative) following an increase in membrane permeability to K^+ via cell surface ion channels in excitable cells

inverse agonist

binds with high affinity to a receptor in its 'resting' state, thus shifting the equilibrium from 'activated' to 'resting' state, and producing the opposite pharmacological effect to an agonist

irreversible competitive antagonist

competes with agonist for the receptor, but the antagonism is insurmountable as the drug only very slowly dissociates from the receptor or in some cases not at all owing to covalent bonding with the receptor

metabolism

the build up, breakdown and excretion of substances in the body; in pharmacology, it is commonly used to refer to the process that is largely responsible for inactivating parent drug molecules by conversion to more polar inactive metabolites ready for elimination by the body

monoamine oxidase (MAO)

an enzyme located on the surface of mitochondria, predominantly in neuronal terminals of aminergic nerves (e.g. noradrenergic nerves); it metabolizes any free cytoplasmic amine (e.g. neurotransmitters such as serotonin, dopamine and norepinephrine) and is a target for the MAO inhibitors

Na$^+$/K$^+$-ATPase

energy-dependent membrane pump that drives Na^+ out of cells and K^+ into cells in order to create an electrochemical gradient

neuromuscular junction

denotes the region of skeletal muscle that receives innervation from somatic nerves

non-competitive antagonist

binds to some point in the sequence of events leading from receptor activation to a pharmacological response and interferes with this process

non-steroidal anti-inflammatory drugs (NSAIDs)

inhibit cyclooxygenase (COX) and prevent the formation of prostaglandins involved in inflammation

parasympathetic nervous system

a subdivision of the autonomic nervous system that utilizes acetylcholine as the principal neurotransmitter secreted at neuroeffector junctions

partial agonist

term used to describe an agonist that produces a submaximal pharmacological response in a given tissue

pharmacodynamics

the study of the biological effect of the drug in vivo and the relationship between drug concentration and pharmacological response

pharmacokinetics

the study of how the body affects drug disposition and provides valuable information concerning the rates of absorption and elimination and the distribution of drug throughout the body

pharmacokinetic antagonist

a chemical that reduces the concentration of drug at receptor sites by promoting the drug's hepatic metabolism, renal excretion or inhibiting absorption from the gastrointestinal tract

phosphodiesterase
family of enzymes that terminate the action of the second messengers cAMP and cGMP

physiological antagonist
a drug that produces a response in a tissue opposite to that of another while not acting at the same receptor, thereby reversing the pharmacological activity of this other substance

pA_2
the negative logarithm of the concentration of antagonist that causes a twofold shift in the dose–response curve to an agonist; it is a measure of antagonist potency calculated from a Schild plot with slope of unity

pK_B
a measure of the potency of an antagonist and is defined as the negative logarithm of the molar concentration of drug that would occupy 50% of the receptors at equilibrium

potency
a measure of the concentration of drug that is pharmacologically active and for agonists is denoted by the EC_{50} or pD_2 (–log EC_{50}) and for antagonists is denoted by pK_B or pA_2

prodrug
pharmacological inactive molecule that is converted by metabolism to a pharmacological active metabolite

receptor
a macromolecule on the surface of the cell or within the cytoplasm or nucleus of a cell that is recognized by a chemical messenger

reversible competitive antagonist
competes with agonist for the receptor, but the antagonism is surmountable and overcome by increasing the concentration of agonist in the vicinity of the receptor

second messenger
endogenous chemical substances (e.g. cAMP, inositol 1,4,5-trisphosphate) generated as a consequence of the activation of a receptor; the second messengers trigger a cascade of events within cells culminating in a pharmacological response

selectivity
the relative potency of a drug for two receptor subtypes (e.g. terfenadine is selective for H_1 but not H2 receptors)

serotonin selective reuptake inhibitors (SSRI)
drugs inhibiting the serotonin (5-hydroxytryptamine) reuptake transporter on serotonergic nerve terminals

spare receptors
the reserve or surplus of receptors in tissues since only a small fraction needs to be occupied by drug in order to elicit a maximal pharmacological response

specificity
the relative potency of drug for two different receptor types (e.g. salbutamol is specific for β-adrenoceptors; pilocarpine is specific for muscarinic receptors)

sympathetic nervous system
a subdivision of the autonomic nervous system with norepinephrine as the principal neurotransmitter secreted at neuroeffector junctions and the hormone epinephrine secreted by the adrenal medulla

therapeutic window
the optimal range of plasma levels for a drug to produce the appropriate pharmacological or therapeutic effect in vivo

uptake 1
a high-affinity transport system for norepinephrine belonging to the family of neurotransmitter transporter proteins in neuronal cells

uptake 2
a low-affinity transport system for amines like epinephrine present in neuronal and non-neuronal cells

volume of distribution
a pharmacokinetic term that is a measure of the amount of drug distributed in the body; it is the theoretical volume into which the total amount of drug in the body is uniformly distributed in order to produce the observed plasma concentration (i.e. it is a hypothetical volume in which the drug would be distributed if its concentration wherever it was distributed was the same as at the sampling site)

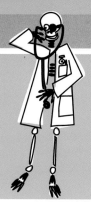

Index